GOOD NIGHT, BRAIN

GOOD NIGHT, BRAIN

7 SLEEP HACKS TO BEAT INSOMNIA: GO TO SLEEP, GET
BACK TO SLEEP, AND STAY ASLEEP

ANTONIA VAN BECKER

GREG LEE

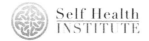

THIS BOOK IS DEDICATED TO:

All our beautiful students and clients who opened their arms to us and shared their vulnerabilities, their voices, and their wisdom. May your light and healing shine brightly in the world.

To Katja Rusanen, Shihan James Henry, Linda Anderson Henry, Chantel Prince, Alisa Clickenger, and our gang of angels, thank you for being your brilliant selves and helping us carry this message into the world.

To our dear daughters, Marika and Nicole (and you, too, Pau!), we are continually brightened by your presence.

To our family and friends, we're so grateful you're here. We love you all.

CONTENTS

GOOD NIGHT, BRAIN

In a dim-lit room, the lights down low,
The candle is lit, and fast turns to slow.
The mind breathes in peace,
The senses smell calm,
The body relaxes as it feels the balm
Of no more news feed, say goodnight to the phone,
Now you are in the sleeping zone.

Good night, noise, good night, light,
Good night, to anything that leads to a fight.
Good night, world, good night, strife,
Good night, to this amazing and wondrous life.
Good night, brain that gives us such chatter,
Good night, lavender that gives us what matters.
Good night, toes all the way to our nose,
Our breathing brings closer what everyone knows,
That the lightness within is what brings us such peace
And gives us good sleep so our healing does increase.

Good night, brain, good night, thinking train.
Good night and sleep tight, while asleep we remain.

INTRODUCTION

Welcome to *Good Night, Brain,* a guide designed to help adults who struggle with insomnia find relief and improve their sleep quality. So many people have sleep issues for a myriad of reasons. Some have a hard time going to sleep because of racing thoughts, regrets of what was left undone, or dwelling on things that happened during the day. Some people wake up many times during the night, whether from the physical issues of having to relieve themselves, old habits and patterns of wakefulness, or an active brain. And while some are able to go back to sleep, others can't stay asleep as long as they would like. Many of these patterns result in feeling tired, depressed, or unmotivated in the morning. If this sounds like your predicament, this book is for you!

Whether you identify with having insomnia, restless sleep, a small bladder, or FOMO (Fear Of Missing Out), which makes going to bed nearly impossible, in *Good Night, Brain*, you'll find many ways to go to sleep, get back to sleep, and stay asleep. And most importantly, you'll find unique methods that work for you and your individual needs.

Everyone is different! Sleep solutions are not one-size-fits-all. Using our processes you get to find what works for you, AND you can change, add, or subtract from your sleep routine so that it adapts as you transform your sleep habits. Once you're able to go to sleep faster, you can focus on staying asleep longer and waking less frequently. Perhaps calming your restless thoughts is of primary importance. You can manage each of these issues and manifest the results you want with just a little creativity, patience, and faith.

Whatever your needs, you can use the various methods in this book (some ancient wisdom, some new thought) to create restful sleep patterns so you can get the rest, healing, and rejuvenation that you need to wake up refreshed, motivated, and at peace.

Sleep is the most important tool in your disease prevention tool kit. Optimal sleep gives you more energy, enhances your immune system, improves memory, increases weight loss, and empowers your brain. The goal, here, is to help you create better sleep patterns and have restful sleep without medication or screen aid, so that you can feel great about yourself and have a healthier and more positive outlook, body, mind, and spirit.

Good Night, Brain, is unique because it offers a holistic approach to tackling insomnia by helping you create sleep solutions that work for you. Unlike other books that focus solely on medical issues or treatments, *Good Night, Brain* addresses the common causes of insomnia and sleep deprivation and helps you create awareness around your own sleep habits and needs. When you understand why you are unable or resistant to going to bed, for example, then it is easier to find a solution that motivates you to go to bed earlier and turn off your light sooner.

By combining awareness, fun, relaxing strategies, and ancient wisdom, this book provides a comprehensive toolkit for overcoming insomnia and achieving restful sleep.

HOW TO USE THIS BOOK

Good Night, Brain, is short and easy to digest so you can read it from cover to cover - if you wish - to get a sense of all the sleep hacks, awareness exercises, and how they can help you sleep.

The first chapter, "Knowing Your Sleep Style," is all about creating awareness of your personal sleep patterns and needs. When you know how you sleep - or don't sleep - and why, then you can more easily change and transform those challenges into the solutions and outcomes you so desire for your own rest and rejuvenation. **Please, please, please use the Good Night, Brain Sleep Log for at least a week or two.** When we used it for the first time, it was shocking in what it revealed about our sleep deprivation. It changed our sleep goals and sleep habits forever.

In "Sleep Hack #1: Creating a Soothing Sleep Environment," you will do a sleep audit to investigate your sleep surroundings and uncover clues about sleep disturbances. Then, you can integrate some of the recommended sleep solutions. Little by little you'll build a firm foundation of restful sleep that you can take with you throughout your life.

"Sleep Hack #2: Establishing a Relaxing Bedtime Routine," is all about what you do before you get in bed and turn out the light. This hack describes the benefits of having a routine around your bedtime so that you can ease into sleep naturally and peacefully.

In "Sleep Hack #3: Limiting Screen Time Before Bed," data shows how many people use screens before bed and how disruptive to sleep it can be. A variety of solutions and strategies are suggested so you can shorten or stop your screen time before bed and get to sleep faster and have a deeper sleep.

In "Sleep Hack #4: Body Relaxation and Energetic Release Techniques," we describe different techniques to relax your body that you can do before bed or in bed (and in the middle of the night), so you can get to sleep or back to sleep quickly and easily! This is so important so that you can wake up in the morning with less pain or absolutely pain free.

"Sleep Hack #5: Using Meditation to Fall Asleep," reinforces how effective meditation can be as a sleep aid, a brain relaxer, and an anxiety calmer! Even if you only meditate for a few moments a day, that's a great start on your meditation journey for more restful sleep.

"Sleep Hack #6: How Conscious Breathing Gets You Into The Sleep Groove," is the biggest transformer of sleep habits that we offer. In this hack, you examine your own breathing patterns to establish your baseline. Then, we talk about how breathing is at the core of all the sleep hacks, and how you can use it to relax your body, calm your brain, deepen your sleep, go to sleep, get back to sleep, and stay asleep.

"In Sleep Hack #7: Cultivating a Positive Sleep Mindset," we create a sleep intention so that all your energy, (body, mind, and spirit) is working toward the same goal. This hack is all about changing how you view sleep, your beliefs about sleep, and to give you some affirmations that will remind you of your newly established positive mindset around sleep.

In the chapter, "Avoiding Sleep Disrupting Activities," we discuss many things that can get in your way of a restful night's sleep: alcohol, stress, mentally triggering activities, excessive exercise, late night eating. Then, we give you ideas and strategies for how to limit or change those activities so that you can develop and strengthen your sleep solutions and change your health and happiness forever.

In the following chapter, "What If It's More Serious?" we look at chronic conditions that could be impacting your sleep. These include nightmares, night terrors, phobias and fears around sleep, darkness, and safety, and how to resolve some of these deeply impactful and traumatic responses to nighttime and bedtime.

The last chapter, "Next Steps," dives into how to set sleep goals, offers you a link to download a cool sleep meditation, and details how to keep in touch for more healing and transformation.

Let's get started and explore how awareness of your sleep style will help you create sleep solutions for whatever is keeping you awake!

FOREWORD

Imagine a moment when the universe orchestrates a connection so serendipitous, it redefines your path in the most unexpected ways. In my case, the magic unfolded in July of 2017. I had put out a call for an accountability buddy in an online program, and Antonia Van Becker responded. The connection was instant, like reuniting with a long-lost friend. Antonia and her husband, Greg Lee, were on a mission to transform sleep for everyone. Leveraging their extensive experience as Master Energetic Healers, they combined deep knowledge in sleep, meditation, energy healing, conscious breathing, and music.

My journey to truly grasp the depth of their work became literal when I flew across the Atlantic from Malaga, Spain, to San Francisco, California. As is often the case for me, getting restful sleep on the plane proved challenging. Surrounded by fellow travelers who seemed to drift off effortlessly, the rhythmic hum of the engines offered a counterpoint to my own wide-eyed wakefulness. I found myself caught between envy and a burgeoning curiosity. What secrets to restful sleep were they privy to that I had missed? This question lingered in my mind as I stepped off the plane, weary and worn.

Arriving at Hummingbird Farm, the sanctuary Antonia and Greg have cultivated, my fatigue from the flight began to dissolve into the serene tranquility of their home. My body and mind started to relax. After a night of deep, restorative sleep, I awoke to a view so beautiful, it seemed like a slice of paradise on Earth. This embodied the holistic well-being that Antonia and Greg nurture.

This personal transformation exemplifies the unique approach *Good Night, Brain* brings to sleep improvement. The book intricately weaves scientific research with holistic practices, offering practical strategies for better sleep and a pathway to a more harmonious, energized existence.

Antonia and Greg's work is a beacon of hope for anyone struggling with insomnia or other sleep issues. They invite us to reframe night as a source of healing and renewal. Readers will be guided through creating a sleep sanctuary, mastering relaxation techniques, cultivating a mindset conducive to rest, and more.

As you delve into this book, approach it with an open mind, ready to be transformed by the wisdom, compassion, and dedication that shine through Antonia and Greg's work. Let their teachings, inspired by their holistic approach and grounded in science, guide you on a transformative exploration of sleep.

Rest is sacred, and *Good Night, Brain* offers a path to rediscovering its power. With Antonia and Greg's guidance, you can unlock a world of restful nights. Imagine waking up feeling rejuvenated, ready to embrace each day with newfound energy. This book has the potential to transform your sleep, and with it, your life.

Dr. Katja Rusanen, Spiritual Counselor

PREFACE

I could hear the ticking of the clock. It sounded unnaturally loud. I opened my eyes to pitch darkness. Greg's soft inhale reminded me where I was. Safe. Home. In bed. And awake. I was tired. It had been a long week, working full time, taking care of the kids, and anxiety pressed my brain awake. My stomach knotted: work stress, too much coffee, family conflicts. I could keep the old panic attacks at bay, but there was worry about work tasks that weren't done, family obligations that made me feel guilty, and wanting to finish a draft of a book that never seemed complete. It all made me feel like I wasn't doing enough. I knew there wasn't much I could do in the middle of the night, but I couldn't shake the dread, so I lay there breathing as the hours went by.

Sleep can be tricky. One-third of adults suffer from insomnia symptoms and up to 22% have insomnia disorder.[1] Occasionally, someone will say, "I sleep like a baby," but most of the time, we hear from clients who have trouble getting to bed or falling asleep, those who wake up and can't get back to sleep because their brain is going

---

1. "What Are Sleep Disorders?" American Psychiatric Association. (2024) www.psychia try.org/patients-families/sleep-disorders/what-are-sleep-disorders

too fast, and those who can't seem to get more than four or five hours of sleep a night.

We've been there, and sometimes, when life gets a little crazy and there's a lot going on, sleep issues can still plague us!

And perhaps you're just like us. We go through periods: maybe there's some drama in the family, or maybe our finances are not as we would like them, or maybe the stuff that's going on in the world is so upsetting that it takes over our peace of mind.

And then it's harder to go to sleep, we toss and turn, uncomfortable, maybe in pain, and when we get up in the morning, we drag and feel uninspired, hoping only to make it through the day.

That's not how we want to live! We want to wake up ready to meet the challenges and triumphs that life has to offer us. We want to embody the equanimity with which a restful sleep can empower us. We want to be happy and healthy.

That's why we wrote this book. To help you with sleep through all different times and aspects of your life. We change as we age, and our patterns and issues change with us. Our bodies change, maybe we have an injury or accident that brings us pain that keeps us awake. Maybe we have a stressful job that feels undoable, and we spend hours at night trying to figure out how to make it work or fuming about why it is the way it is. Perhaps we have a young child who doesn't sleep well.

Everyone is an individual, and we go through our life changes in our own way. *Good Night, Brain* will give you sleep solutions that you can use no matter where you are in life and what is going on for you. You'll be able to create your own sleep sanctuary, so you feel safe and able to relax. From there, you can build other sleep skills as your needs change.

I've always been a morning person. I would get up early and go running when I was a teenager or go to a 5:00 or 6:00 a.m. job when I got older. My sleep trouble started when I started to go to bed later and later. There was just so much to do - whether that was in college and socializing til late on the weekends (with Greg when we were dating!) and then during the week having to stay up late to get my homework done, so I could never get to bed before 2:00 a.m.! And because I could never sleep in, I felt exhausted most of the time.

This exhaustion (and ACEs, which we'll talk about later) led to my getting bronchitis and pneumonia on a regular basis until I realized that getting regular sleep was an important factor in repairing my health. This took years, and we don't want it to take that long for you. Whatever your cause for not sleeping, and however it is affecting your mental or physical health, we want this book to be the shortcut to your sleep solutions.

What we know for sure is that it doesn't need to be complicated. It may take practice, it may take some time, it may take shifting something in your schedule – or in your brain – but you too can get restful sleep.

Just as we are all unique, we all have different sleep issues. When I was a kid, I had panic attacks during the night. At the time I didn't understand what they were, but waking up sweating and shaking was upsetting, and I lost a lot of sleep during those times.

Later, in my young adult years, there was a time when using alcohol, caffeine, and other recreational drugs highly interfered with my sleep, leaving me with a legacy of doubting that I could sleep well. Those habits also triggered the old panic attacks and further undermined my sleep confidence.

It wasn't until Greg and I escaped the corporate world, and started doing energetic healing that we realized the complexity of sleep disorders. We realized that many of the core issues that create sleep issues reside in the adverse experiences that we've had. Those adverse experiences can lead to anxiety, fear, guilt, anger and the associated panic, dread, rage, insomnia, and chronic illness. But often it's not obvious! That's why, despite the medical community knowing that ACEs (Adverse Childhood Experiences) have an outsized negative effect on people's health and happiness across a lifetime, there is no cure for it once it has happened.

And this is where our big 'Ah Ha' came in. CoreTalk™, the energetic healing that we had been doing for years, relieved our ACEs. When we learned to work with the body's innate healing system, we could heal the fear or anger or guilt and that allowed us to go back to sleep faster and easier.

What I didn't realize when I was in grade school is that I was stressed out by my parents' constant arguing and drinking, and that's what caused my panic attacks in the middle of the night. Later, when my brother's mental illness became more pronounced, I felt (subconsciously at the time) that I had to work hard to NOT be like him: to be very functional, to hold the family together when it was falling apart, and to make sure everyone was alright. I had a lot of balls in the air, and it kept me awake many nights.

And then, as our CoreTalk healing business grew from one-on-one clinical work to working with groups online (even before the pandemic), I wanted to create a training that was foundational for everyone's health. It quickly became obvious that the most important aspect of our lives, the one thing that impacted us more than anything else, was sleep.

Back then, when I created that first online sleep training to help people beat insomnia (and when I met Katja), it had amazing results. The participants turned off their TVs, they went to bed earlier, and slept longer. They felt better and were happier during the day and were inspired to do their life's work, whatever that was.

Now, in *Good Night, Brain*, we hope to give you similar results. We believe that by applying some, or many, of these techniques and processes in your life, you will build your sleep confidence. You can create a place in your home and in your brain where you can sleep long and sound, where you fall back asleep easily, and where you'll wake up refreshed.

KNOWING YOUR SLEEP STYLE

WHAT IS YOUR SLEEP STYLE? When do you like to sleep? How much sleep do you need? What are your sleep patterns, issues, and beliefs? Knowing all about your habits around sleep is pivotal to being able to create sleep solutions that are just right for you. This awareness will make it so much easier to identify your needs and put your optimal solutions into place. Then you can shift your priorities when your needs shift as you create more and better sleep for yourself.

This chapter is about getting to know yourself and how and why you sleep or don't sleep well. It also includes a sleep log to document how much sleep you're actually getting in order to give you a realistic starting place for your sleep goals. Answering each of the questions posed in this chapter will give you an overall awareness of your personal sleep profile. You may be surprised at how complex some of these issues are and why they're still an issue! If it was easy, you would have fixed it already, right? Give yourself some love that you are doing this very interesting investigation for and about yourself right here, right now. Let's jump in!

ARE YOU A MORNING OR NIGHT PERSON?

Answer the following questions by looking back over your entire life's sleep patterns up to the present day. Look at how you slept when you were a kid. Many times, those were your natural sleep patterns, for example, if you always woke up early. Also, take into consideration if you stayed up late (or got up early) as a result of a job or extra study-ing, not because of natural desire. Important to note is how your patterns changed over the years, and whether there was a pattern of getting up early or staying up late.

And, even if you know you're a morning or a night person, take a moment to check the list below to see if anything has changed or, if underneath long held habits and beliefs, your body might desire a different pattern.

- Did/Do you often go to bed early?
- Did/Do you fall asleep easily at night?
- What time did you wake up as a kid?
- Did you choose a job or career that required early mornings?
- Did/Do you often go to bed late?
- Is it hard to go to sleep early?
- Did/Do you love to sleep in?
- Was/Is it hard to wake up early?
- Did you choose a career that required late nights?

Get a sense of when you get your best sleep and how you feel in the morning. Feeling vibrant and ready to go in the morning is a clue that you've gotten the sleep you need on a consistent basis.

HOW MUCH SLEEP DO YOU NEED?

Several years ago, I was always tired, my mind would blank out trying to remember things, and I got grumpy a lot. At that time, I was getting some music theory coaching, and my mentor had me keep a sleep log.

He asked me to think about how much sleep I ideally wanted. At that time, I rarely got more than six hours, but I remembered how good I felt after getting eight hours a night.

So, I tracked my hours for a week. I was shocked. Because I was only getting 5-6 hours of sleep a night, by the end of the first week's tally, I was down 12 hours to my goal of 8 hours a night. I had a sleep deficit I wasn't able to regain. That was when I decided that I needed to change my sleep habits.

THE GOOD NIGHT, BRAIN SLEEP LOG

Using the Good Night, Brain Sleep Log at the end of this chapter to log your sleep hours and quality will give you a good overview of how much sleep you're getting and what your sleep patterns are.

Studies show that 30% of Americans get less than 6.5 hours sleep and are sleep deprived.[1] I was one of them. Are you?

By using the sleep log, I became more aware of my sleep patterns, and I realized that when I was very tired, I would hit my head. Do you have something that happens when you're tired? Do you trip or drop things? Do you get frustrated easily? Do you eat more to keep your energy up? Physical and mental reaction time also goes down when you're tired, so you have to be more careful when driving a car or operating heavy machinery!

The Mayo Clinic recommends seven or more hours of sleep per night for adults 18 years of age or older.[2]

Look at your habits and remember when you felt the best and how many hours of sleep you were getting. If you dowse or muscle test, do so to ask your body how many hours of sleep it wants to get each night. You may be surprised at the answer. (If you want to learn how

---

1. "Sleep and Sleep Disorders: Data and Statistics" Centers for Disease Control and Prevention. (2017) www.cdc.gov/sleep/data-research/facts-stats/adults-sleep-facts-and-stats.html
2. "How Many Hours of Sleep Are Enough?" Mayo Clinic (2024) www.mayoclinic.org/healthy-lifestyle/adult-health/expert-answers/how-many-hours-of-sleep-are-enough/faq-20057898

to dowse or muscle test, email us at support@selfhealthinstitute.com. We love to teach people how to talk to their body to find out how much sleep it needs!) If you don't muscle test, you can use your intuition to get the answer. If you're muscle testing, make sure you're not talking to your brain! Your brain might want you to stay up late to get stuff done!

Write down the answer you get from your body.

I would like to get _____ hours of sleep every night.

WHAT ARE YOUR SLEEP PATTERNS AND ISSUES?

All of us have different patterns of sleep and wakefulness. Being aware of those patterns can help you focus on and prioritize which patterns you would like to change.

Going to Sleep

- Is it hard to make yourself go to bed or turn off the light?
- Is it hard to go to sleep?
- Does it take longer to go to sleep than you wish?
- Do you have racing thoughts or anxiety?
- Do you have restless leg syndrome?
- Do you have pain?
- Does anyone in your household wake you up when you're trying to go to sleep?
- Do you have to take a sleep aid to go to sleep?
- Do you always want to watch one more episode because then you can fall asleep easier?
- Do you go to sleep with the TV on?

Getting Back to Sleep

- Is it hard to go back to sleep?
- Do you have racing thoughts or anxiety?

- Do you have restless leg syndrome?
- Do you have pain?
- Are you sometimes/often too hot or cold?
- Are you sometimes/often thirsty or hungry?
- Are you sometimes/often too full or intoxicated?

Staying Asleep

- Do you have to get up to relieve yourself many times during the night?
- Do you often wake up with bad dreams or racing thoughts?
- Do you often wake up at a certain time of night?
- Do you only get a few hours of sleep at a time?
- Do you get up in the night because of an animal or person?
- Does your sleep partner snore or have sleep issues that wake you up?

You may want to evaluate your sleep patterns and issues over several weeks as circumstances in your life will vary. Use the following Good Night, Brain Sleep Log to track your progress.

After your evaluation, do you have a sense of what your sleep issues are? It's a good idea to tackle just one or two sleep issues at a time so you can see what works for you before you move on to the next issue.

For the ease of prioritization, decide: is the first issue I want to work on about going to sleep, getting back to sleep, or staying asleep? Once you have decided that, narrow your focus to one of your issues. Then, move ahead to find solutions and strategies for that issue in the Sleep Hacks.

The sleep issue I want to work on first is

BELIEFS AND EMOTIONAL SETTINGS AROUND SLEEP

Wow! We're cookin' with gas now!

And, we're going deep! This is important so we can discover the issues underlying the lack of optimal sleep. Now that we've examined the more surface or physical habits of sleep, we also want to delve into what is going on inside of us on the mental and emotional level. This means looking at what sleep means or feels like to us when we're not sleeping or when we're trying to sleep.

How many negative thought patterns or beliefs are playing underneath your thoughts, or perhaps right on the surface? Thoughts like "I can't do that," "That's too scary," or "Why bother, it's never going to work," are often going through our minds quickly without our conscious awareness. What thoughts can you catch in your mind? Those negative thoughts can stop you from taking actions that increase your happiness, opportunities, and overall well-being.

Becoming aware of and changing those negative beliefs or thought patterns are key to creating a mental environment that is conducive to long and restful sleep and being able to overcome insomnia. Research has shown that individuals with a positive outlook on sleep are more likely to experience better sleep quality and duration compared to those with negative sleep beliefs.

SOME OF THE THOUGHTS AND BELIEFS ABOUT SLEEP COULD BE:

- I'm a light sleeper and wake up easily.
- I can only sleep a couple hours at a time.
- I don't want to go to bed because I'll miss something.
- Going to bed early feels like giving up on my To Do List.
- Sleep is a waste of time.
- I should be working and not sleeping.
- I don't want to go to bed because I have nightmares.
- It's not safe to fall asleep.

- It's scary to be in the dark.
- If I go to bed too early, I won't be able to go to sleep (or get back to sleep).
- I feel lazy if I give myself a full night's sleep
- I need to stay up late to get the important stuff done.
- I'll sleep when I die.
- I can't sleep alone.
- I need complete darkness and quiet to fall asleep
- I need a sleep aid to fall asleep
- I need the TV on to fall asleep

These thoughts, emotions and beliefs can influence us short or long term: either for one night or for a lifetime.

We've seen many clients develop FOMO (Fear Of Missing Out) when they were young. They never wanted to go to bed because they would miss out on the fun or various experiences the older kids or parents were having. They end up always wishing they could stay up later, and so when they have the freedom to choose, they stay up later because they can. This can develop into a lifelong habit of always wanting to watch one more episode or one more training, and to avoid going to sleep for whatever reason.

Similarly, a short-term example is when I have an early alarm or a big project due the next morning. I really want to have a good sleep so I can be refreshed. That's when I worry that I'll get the amount of sleep I want. I wake up, once, twice, three times, looking at my phone to see what time it is and how much longer I have to sleep. Looking at the phone's blue light wakes my brain just a little more, and then, it kicks my brain into thinking. This sets the cycle of wakefulness until I look at my clock again. This short term – or one night pattern of waking up – can cause slowness or a foggy brain the next day right when you want to be refreshed. It is definitely not optimal, especially if it happens on a regular basis.

Short (and long) term sleep issues may also be related to other issues in your life: being worried about whether you're good or worthy enough, feeling like you always have to be prepared to avoid getting into trouble or being wrong or criticized, or being vigilant so you don't get hurt. We look at some of these related issues in the chapter called, "What If It's More Serious." And while we don't deal with how to heal those issues in this book, in our clinical work at Self Health Institute, we love helping people feel calm and confident and living in their zone of genius. This is our jam, what we excel at and love to do.

WHAT ARE YOUR BELIEFS ABOUT SLEEP?

The essential ingredient in combating both of these short and long term sleep issues is to understand your unique emotional settings and beliefs around sleep. Give yourself some love around this because you probably have had these same beliefs for a long time, and you came by them righteously! They may have been from experiences when you were very young. Now, you get to change that and create the life and sleep that you want, starting right now.

Shifting your perspective from viewing sleep as a battleground or source of frustration, to seeing sleep as a natural and essential part of life is key to being able to adopt a new sleep pattern or habit. Embrace the idea that your body knows how to sleep and trust in its ability to rest and rejuvenate during the night. By letting go of worries and fears about sleep, you can create space for relaxation and allow sleep to unfold naturally.

Begin listing your sleep beliefs. Allow yourself to do this over time. It is very interesting how more sleep beliefs may unfold as you go through the Sleep Hacks. This is all part of discovering the layers of feelings, thoughts, and beliefs you have around sleep.

In "Sleep Hack #7: Cultivating a Positive Sleep Mindset," you'll create a Sleep Intention that you can use to counter your most detrimental belief around sleep.

YOUR BELIEFS AND EMOTIONAL SETTINGS AROUND SLEEP

_____

_____

_____

_____

_____

_____

_____

_____

_____

_____

GOOD NIGHT, BRAIN SLEEP LOG

The Good Night, Brain Sleep Log, is a valuable tool for tracking the amount of sleep you get and your sleep patterns. Tracking your sleep every night can be a truly enlightening experience, especially if you know you're not getting enough sleep. By consistently using the Sleep Log, you can gain insight into your sleep habits, identify trends or patterns, and make informed adjustments to optimize your sleep quality. Let's explore how to use the Good Night, Brain Sleep Log to support your journey to better sleep.

USING THE GOOD NIGHT, BRAIN SLEEP LOG

Bedtime: Record the time you go to bed each night. This can help you become aware of how certain activities may impact your ability to get more sleep, so you can establish a more consistent bedtime if you wish.

Wake-Up Time: Note the time you wake up each morning. Tracking your wake-up time can help you identify trends in your sleep duration and assess your own ease of falling back to sleep. If you use an alarm to wake up for work, take note of when you wake up on non-workdays.

Sleep Duration: Calculate the total duration of your sleep each night, from the time you go to bed to the time you wake up. Note times when you're awake during the night and subtract that amount. (However, don't stress in the middle of the night thinking about it!)

Sleep Quality: Rate the quality of your sleep each night on a scale of 1 to 10, with 1 being poor and 10 being excellent. Consider factors such as how easily you fell asleep, the depth of your sleep, how many times you woke up, and how rested you felt upon waking.

Notes: Make note of any factors that may have influenced your sleep quality, such as room temperature, lighting, noise, stress levels, physical discomfort, or other factors. Reflect on whether limiting screen time, practicing relaxation techniques, and avoiding caffeine or alcohol in the hours leading up to bedtime had a positive impact.

TIPS FOR USING THE GOOD NIGHT, BRAIN SLEEP LOG

Be Consistent: Make a commitment to fill out the Sleep Log for at least a week, ideally right before bedtime and upon waking in the morning. Consistency is your key to gaining meaningful insights into your sleep patterns.

Be Honest: Be honest and accurate when you write down your findings, even if the information may not reflect positively on your sleep habits. The Sleep Log is a tool for self-awareness and improvement, and honest feedback is essential for making meaningful changes. Plus, today is a new day to make the changes you wish for! It doesn't matter when you make your desired improvements, what's important is that you're doing it now!!

Review Regularly: Take time to review your Sleep Log regularly to identify trends or patterns in your sleep habits. Look for correlations between your sleep quality and factors such as bedtime routines, environmental conditions, daily habits, and peace of mind during the day. Notice how caffeine, alcohol, food, and screen time affect your ability to experience a good sleep. Check out the chapter, "Avoiding Sleep Disrupting Activities," for more information.

Adjust as Needed: Use the insights gained from your Sleep Log to make informed adjustments to your sleep habits and bedtime routines. Experiment with these adjustments and monitor the impact on your sleep quality over time.

And, most importantly, have fun! This is an interesting experiment about your life and habits! What can this show you about your own conceptions, beliefs and patterns about sleep? What will this reveal about your life and how you live it? How can you use this to change some old habits and establish new, more nurturing ones?

This is all about you taking care of you. This is about you giving yourself the gift of self-care. This is the most important gift you can give yourself. Your current and future self will thank you!

You can download your gift of the Good Night, Brain Sleep Log, along with a Sleep Meditation here:

www.selfhealthinstitute.com/sleepgifts

By using this sleep log and reflecting on your sleep habits, you've taken an important step toward improving your sleep quality and overcoming insomnia. With dedication and persistence, you can achieve restful nights and wake up feeling refreshed and energized. Sweet dreams!

WHAT YOU'LL GET FROM KNOWING YOUR SLEEP STYLE

Discovering your sleep patterns, issues, and beliefs can be an incredibly transformational journey. You're diving into some core issues and habits that you may have had for a long time and that have impacted you profoundly. Knowing your own unique patterns, issues, and beliefs is the key to creating a solution that gives you, not only more rest and rejuvenation, but also the fuel to boost your self-esteem, confidence, and allow your dreams to take flight.

Interestingly, once you decide to take action to clear up your concerns around sleep, several issues may clear up on their own. We look at different ways to do that in the chapter, "What If It's More Serious?"

Let's move on to Sleep Hack #1 and create your beautiful, soothing sleep sanctuary.

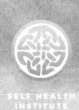

SLEEP LOG

TOTAL HOURS SLEEP THIS WEEK:

DATE:

- I went to bed at _____ I woke up at_____
  Total hours sleep_____
- My quality of sleep was (restful, wakeful, etc.)
  _____
- I woke up _____ times during the night and
  stayed awake for_____
- Factors that might have influenced my sleep
  _____

DATE:

- I went to bed at _____ I woke up at_____
  Total hours sleep_____
- My quality of sleep was (restful, wakeful, etc.)
  _____
- I woke up _____ times during the night and
  stayed awake for_____
- Factors that might have influenced my sleep
  _____

DATE:

- I went to bed at _____ I woke up at_____
  Total hours sleep_____
- My quality of sleep was (restful, wakeful, etc.)
  _____
- I woke up _____ times during the night and
  stayed awake for_____
- Factors that might have influenced my sleep
  _____

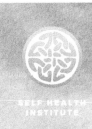

GOOD NIGHT, BRAIN

ANTONIA VAN BECKER AND GREG LEE

DATE:

- I went to bed at _____ I woke up at _____
  Total hours sleep_____
- My quality of sleep was (restful, wakeful, etc.)
  _____
- I woke up _____ times during the night and
  stayed awake for_____
- Factors that might have influenced my sleep
  _____

DATE:

- I went to bed at _____ I woke up at _____
  Total hours sleep_____
- My quality of sleep was (restful, wakeful, etc.)
  _____
- I woke up _____ times during the night and
  stayed awake for_____
- Factors that might have influenced my sleep
  _____

DATE:

- I went to bed at _____ I woke up at_____
  Total hours sleep_____
- My quality of sleep was (restful, wakeful, etc.)
  _____
- I woke up _____ times during the night and
  stayed awake for_____
- Factors that might have influenced my sleep
  _____

DATE:

- I went to bed at _____ I woke up at_____
  Total hours sleep_____
- My quality of sleep was (restful, wakeful, etc.)
  _____
- I woke up _____ times during the night and
  stayed awake for_____
- Factors that might have influenced my sleep
  _____

SLEEP HACK #1: CREATING A SOOTHING SLEEP SANCTUARY

In a dim-lit room, the lights down low,
The candle is lit and fast turns to slow.

THE IMPORTANCE of creating a soothing sleep sanctuary for improving sleep quality cannot be understated. It's all about having a peaceful and safe atmosphere to signal to your brain that it's time to unwind. This chapter will explore how environmental factors such as temperature, lighting, and noise impact sleep quality, and we'll touch on how to optimize our environment for better sleep. We'll conduct a bedroom audit to help you identify what you can change for a more positive sleep experience. We'll also look at other factors that impact our sleep quality, including the sleep habits of the people and animals we sleep with.

Before we begin looking at the external factors that create a soothing sleep environment, let's have a word about your internal environment and how you think and feel about where you're sleeping. Creating a sleep sanctuary begins in your brain and body. If you're thinking or feeling that you're not safe, it will be difficult to feel like you're in a sanctuary where you can fall asleep in peace.

LET'S TALK ABOUT YOUR BRAIN

The brain is wired to keep you safe. According to neuropsychologist, Dr. Rick Hanson, "The mind is like Velcro for negative experiences and Teflon for positive ones." In other words, we hold on to bad experiences, and diminish (or push away) positive experiences so that we can see anything dangerous that's coming our way and survive! YIKES! This is how we're wired. So in order to create a sleep sanctuary, we must look at how we think and feel about where we're sleeping, how comfortable we are in our surroundings, and if we feel safe with the people around us.

We began to look at our emotional settings and beliefs around sleep in the last chapter. We want to go a little deeper here to uncover some, possibly subconscious, issues around sleep. If you feel like you did enough in the last chapter, great! You can move ahead to the section on What Does Your Sleep Sanctuary Look and Feel Like?

If we've had or are having negative experiences in the bedroom and/or at night, it will be very difficult to tell the brain that this is a safe place to relax and go to sleep. This is the foundation for your sleep sanctuary - the fundamental need to feel safe (and happy is a plus) in your sleep environment.

Think about the following questions with regard to your experiences around sleep. Journal about them if you like.

- Do you feel safe in your bedroom?
- Do you like being in your bedroom?
- Have you had negative experiences in a bedroom that might contribute to your not feeling safe?
- Have you had multiple experiences over time in a bedroom that might contribute to your not feeling safe?
- Are you afraid of the dark?
- Are there monsters in the closet or under the bed?

When you don't feel safe, there's a good chance you'll go into Fight and Flight or Sympathetic Mode when you're in the bedroom or in bed. Once in this hyper-aware or hyper-vigilant mode, your body is releasing catecholamines (natural steroids) that are designed to keep you awake so that you can watch for danger.

It's natural that if you've had difficult experiences in a bedroom, that you would feel uncomfortable or unsafe in that environment again. And, interestingly, because no one really wants to think about these difficult experiences, we may have shifted our internal thoughts away from the difficult experiences and to something about not wanting to go to bed or being a light sleeper. And that all makes sense.

However, in order to get to the core of the issue of our sleep problem, we want to acknowledge what the core problem may be and look for solutions from there. We want to be able to shift that feeling of vigilance, fear, or lack of safety to one of security and comfort.

And, most importantly right now: if you don't feel safe because of a person or a situation in your life, you'll want to make a change as soon as possible. It is your right to feel safe.

If you had difficult experiences in the past, but you're safe now, AND you still feel unsafe, there are ways to heal those feelings so that you can feel safe.

This internal understanding of how our brain works and how that is reflected into our bodies will revolutionize your ability to heal what is creating the stress and fear that might be keeping you awake or waking you up.

We look to our body's healing ability in our innate healing system, the meridians and the chakras, to help us heal these adverse experiences that have happened or are still happening. Look to the last chapter in this book, "What If It's More Serious," to see solutions for these sleep safety issues.

Becoming aware of how you think and feel about where you're sleeping is pivotal to understanding, healing, and transforming your emotions, thoughts, and beliefs around your ability to feel safe and sleep well. To this end, in Sleep Hack #7, we will create a Sleep Intention, designed to change any negative beliefs or emotional settings around sleep (including those around being safe). You get to feel safe! You get to be in a place where you ARE safe!

Your ability to feel safe in your bedroom is essential to getting the quality sleep you need. You can make the changes and do the healing you need in order to feel safe, and this will reflect throughout your life, into every aspect of your health, wealth, and well-being.

Wow! Good job looking at the very internal aspect of creating a Sleep Sanctuary. Now, how do you want your Sleep Sanctuary to look and feel on a more external level? Let's look at how to make our bedroom so cozy and alluring that it draws us into sleep.

WHAT DOES YOUR SLEEP SANCTUARY LOOK AND FEEL LIKE?

Everyone wants a bedroom that we love to be in physically, emotionally, and spiritually. The room can be any shape or size, but what matters is that you have things you love or that are important to you in it. Maybe that includes pictures of loved ones, your favorite books, instruments, artwork or mementos from special times in your life. Many people also love to have spiritual texts, symbols, or artwork in their room to remind them of their connection to love, God, and the universe. Anything that reminds you of safe, warm, and happy times are perfect to have in your bedroom.

When I was in grade school, I had a bedroom all to myself. My mom even let me paint it pink for my birthday when I was eight. I covered one wall with huge posters of lions and tigers (yes, I still watch cat videos). On another wall was a floor to ceiling bookcase filled with children's and young adult books. I had a desk under the window on which I painted a princess girl with long curly locks. I was in heaven. I spent a lot of time in my room. It was my sanctuary.

Use joy, intuition, and a sense of play to create your own beautiful space! If you prefer a clear visual field, keep your belongings sparse so you can enjoy and relax into your surroundings. If you like more reminders of your adventures, then have more belongings on display.

What's important is that you create a space that's right for you and makes you happy. It doesn't have to be fancy, just comfortable so you can relax into it. When Greg and I moved in together, we had a lot of thrift store items that worked for us.

Another dimension of creating your sleep sanctuary is to consider the light. Use candles, nightlights, or dimmable (or three-way) bedside lamps with warm-toned bulbs to create a calming and low light ambiance.

Look for sheets, blankets, and throws for your bed that help you maintain your ideal temperature AND feel and look the way you want them to. You want to have the "I'm so happy to be here" feeling when you climb into bed!

You get to create a sleep sanctuary that's perfect for you! Yours will be unique. **This is a powerful act of self-care.** If you share a room, then some compromise may be necessary, but making subtle changes can make all the difference, and your partner may not even notice!

Now that we've touched on how our sleep sanctuary looks and feels, let's look at what we can do with the physical aspect of our bedrooms to make a more conducive sleep environment.

We'll start by conducting a bedroom audit to help you identify what you can change for a more positive sleep experience.

CONDUCTING A BEDROOM AUDIT

Take a proactive approach to optimizing your sleep environment by conducting a thorough audit of your bedroom. As you read through each of the following sections, go through your bedroom to check for potential issues. Do the bedroom audit at night so you can simulate your real sleep experience. Identify potential sleep disruptors such as lights, noise, and temperature issues. Write the issues down or correct them on the spot.

When we talk about the animals and people we sleep with, the changes may be harder to make, but if they are seriously impacting your quality of sleep and life, you may have to use your imagination to come up with some creative solutions.

LIGHTING

Light exposure, particularly in the evening, can affect your circadian rhythm and melatonin production, the hormone that regulates sleep-wake cycles. These Circadian rhythms – our body clock – are an internal 24-hour cycle in which our sleep, hunger, and thirst, ebb and flow with the natural cycles of the sun and the temperatures around us.

It's natural that when the sun and the temperature go down, we start producing the hormone melatonin, and we begin to wind down and get tired. When the sun comes up, and we open our eyes to the light, our bodies begin producing serotonin, a neurotransmitter that regulates our anxiety, happiness, and moods.

So, in order to get optimal sleep, we must help the body see that it's getting dark in order to trigger the sleep portion of the circadian rhythm and the production of melatonin.

That's why it's important for us to look at how many light sources we have in our bedrooms.

The more light sources we have, the more incorrect signals we are sending to our bodies about sleep. We get rid of the light sources, and then our bodies believe that it's time to sleep.

Look around your bedroom. (It works best in the dark.) How many lights do you see? Count them. Do you have a light shining in your window? Or a skylight where a street light shines through? Do you have an alarm clock with a bright dial or a tv that glows, or computer lights?

I have a work desk in my bedroom, and I counted 7 lights JUST from the desk area. Computers, phones, internet hotspot, and surge protectors, all have LEDS that emit light. It's amazing how much light is glowing in our rooms!

Cover LEDS with blue (or masking) tape. Get a different alarm clock with a dimmable dial. Shut the TV off and put it in a cabinet or cover it with a scarf, throw, or blanket. Put the computer in a different room or cover with a cloth. You can always cover lights with socks or tape when nothing else works! Unplug electronics and internet at night.

Invest in blackout curtains or shades to block out external light sources through the windows or skylight.

For people with nightmares or night terrors, complete darkness can be a problem. No worries! A nightlight is very helpful, especially if the light is diffuse. We talk more about this issue in the chapter entitled, "What If It's More Serious?"

We will also talk about using phones or tablets right before bed, and the negative effect that can have on your sleep in "Sleep Hack #3: Limiting Screen Time Before Bed."

TEMPERATURE

The temperature of your sleep environment plays a significant role in your ability to fall asleep and stay asleep. The National Sleep Foundation recommends that you keep your bedroom slightly cool, around 65 degrees Fahrenheit (15-19 degrees Celsius) to promote better sleep.[1]

Experiment with adjusting your thermostat to find the optimal room temperature for your sleep needs.

Also, what you wear or don't wear to bed is going to influence your internal temperature. as will the weight and number of your blankets. While this might sound elementary, have some fun changing up your blankets and pajamas as the weather and seasons change.

Some people also love to sleep with the window open no matter what the temperature is outside. This can be very refreshing and promote deep sleep, as long as outside noise doesn't become a problem.

---

1. "10 Tips for a Better Night's Sleep" National Sleep Foundation (2024) www.thensf. org/sleep-tips/

NOISE

Noise pollution can disrupt your sleep and lead to fragmented sleep patterns. Identify sources of noise in your bedroom and take steps to minimize or eliminate them. Phones ringing, alarms going off, computers beeping, and household utilities running can all keep you awake or wake you up.

Sudden noise can also cause a fear or panic response that can keep you awake long after the noise has stopped.

Therefore, the best options are to keep computers or phones out of the bedroom or shut off. Be sure to run laundry or dishes well before bed. If you can't stop the noise from happening (like street or roommate noise), minimize noise disturbances by using earplugs, fans, or soundproofing measures to create a quieter sleep environment. You can also employ white noise machines or other electronic devices that can deliver nature or water sounds to mask external noise.

WHO DO YOU SLEEP WITH?

Of all the possible sleep disturbances, this is the most tricky and close to the heart. We're not here to tell you to make any specific decisions, only to give you information so you can do what is best for you.

ANIMALS

As an animal lover, I have lived and slept with animals my entire life. When I was young, the dog and cat got most of the room in the bed, but I never minded. They gave me a sense of security and love that was very important to me.

We still love our animals, but now we have a few more boundaries. That said, whatever works for you is great! It's only when the cat keeps waking you up or the dog snores, that you may want to rethink your sleeping arrangements.

Many people allow their pets on the bed until lights out and then ask them to get in their own beds. There are many types and styles of animal beds to keep our furry family safe and warm if you would like to make this move. There may be some initial grumbling, but they do get used to it, and many times they relish having their own space.

If a cat is continually waking you up at night (after all they are nocturnal), there are various methods you can use to modulate these interruptions. Often, we'll invite our cat outside or for a playtime before bed. This gives him some exercise and play so he can easily go to sleep when we go to sleep. Since cats sleep 16-20 hours a day, often she doesn't wake up until early morning.

We're all creatures of habit, and we may need to become more aware of our animals' sleep habits so that we can all enjoy a better night's sleep.

PEOPLE

Decisions around changing sleeping habits can be fraught with emotions. However, decisions that positively impact sleep can also result in happier, more tranquil relationships and life.

If you have a loved one that snores, needs equipment to sleep, or is up and down during the night, and they are negatively affecting your mental or physical health, you may have to consider different sleeping arrangements. We've known many couples who sleep separately and yet maintain loving and intimate relationships. Some couples sleep separately on certain nights and not others. Many couples would never think of sleeping separately, no matter what the challenges are.

Some couples have very specific boundaries around when they go to sleep or wake up. When these boundaries are made and maintained in a loving manner, they can be very helpful to contribute to your sleep sanctuary. Those boundaries may also help your partner or other people in the household get better sleep. When you do what is best for you, it's best for everyone.

Where and who you sleep with is a very personal decision to make, but one we brought up here just to show the many possibilities that exist to get the sleep you need. Again, creativity can bring in fun, peace, and lasting solutions.

MAKE CREATING YOUR SLEEP SANCTUARY FUN

Have fun creating a sleep sanctuary so you look forward to going to bed! We spend about a third of our lives in bed, so we might as well make the most of it! Having an optimal sleep environment tailored to your needs and preferences will set the stage for your beautiful night's sleep.

SLEEP HACK #2: ESTABLISHING A RELAXING BEDTIME ROUTINE

The mind breathes in peace
The senses smell calm

TO ACHIEVE RESTFUL SLEEP, establishing a calming bedtime routine is essential. In this Sleep Hack, we'll explore the importance of a consistent bedtime routine in signaling to your brain that it's time to wind down and prepare for sleep. Reading, gentle stretching, or listening to calming music can help you say "goodnight" to your worries and thoughts, easing your mind into a state of relaxation.

According to the American Academy of Sleep Medicine, implementing a bedtime routine consisting of calming activities and relaxation techniques significantly improved sleep quality and reduced symptoms of insomnia.[1]

Completing your routine every night reinforces your body's natural sleep-wake cycle, making it easier to fall asleep and wake up feeling refreshed. Let's explore how to establish a bedtime routine that sets the stage for a restful night's sleep.

---

1. "Healthy Sleep Habits" American Academy of Sleep Medicine (2024) https://sleeped ucation.org/healthy-sleep/healthy-sleep-habits/

YOU GET TO HAVE IT YOUR WAY

Your bedtime routine includes everything you do BEFORE you get in bed and turn out the light. This is not a one-size-fits-all routine. You get to establish a pattern that works the best for you!

There are many choices to explore so you can find the routine that nourishes and sends you into a deep, restful sleep. As you look at all the possibilities we've outlined below, you may not come upon the perfect routine all at once, but rather piece by piece as you find the elements that are truly comforting and relaxing for you. This is, after all, for YOU. You are creating a very important self-care routine that will affect your health and happiness for a long time to come!

Listed below are elements of a relaxing bedtime routine. Pick out a few elements that call to you, and then try others to find the right fit. If you already have a bedtime routine, evaluate how it is working for you, and then see what you might add or subtract to make it more effective.

Importantly, don't let your bedtime routine turn into something that keeps you up! This routine is to enable you to go to bed so you can get the amount of sleep you need. Use the number of hours you want to sleep each night in calculating your bedtime based on when you have to get up.

Your Sleep Intention is to get YOUR optimal number of hours of sleep!

And don't forget to be forgiving of yourself if you don't always hit your sleep numbers or complete your routine. We aren't perfect, but the continued intention to meet your goals will help you reach them one day at a time. Let this be relaxing and exactly right for you.

BEDTIME READING

Do you have a genre of books that you love to read: maybe mysteries, non-fiction, or perhaps spiritual? How do they make you feel? What you read before you go to bed impacts what you're thinking about before you sleep and dream. Discover how you want to feel as you go to sleep and read something that reflects and deepens that feeling. In other words, pay attention to what effect reading has on you.

Do you fall asleep quickly when you start to read? Great! Set your number of pages to a very few, so you can put the book down and turn the light off before you fall asleep. Does reading stimulate you? If so, put a firm limit on your number of pages, so you don't stay up too late! Or look at a different type of reading material that may have a more soothing effect at bedtime.

And, just as a reminder, you'll want to read a physical book, not a digital one. Have fun finding that hard copy book that will sooth you into a beautiful night's rest. Maybe it's something completely different than your usual: try poems, essays, or spiritual texts! Whatever relaxes you will help you fall asleep quickly and easily.

JOURNALING

Many people love to have a gratitude journal by their bedside to write about all the things they were grateful for that day. Others love to take a few minutes to jot down thoughts, worries, or reflections. Others take an inventory of what happened that day, and what they wished they had done differently. Some people write down everything they need to do the next day, so they don't have to think about it during the night.

Be aware of the effect these different types of journaling have on you. Does thinking about what you have to do the next day stimulate your brain, making it harder to sleep? Some people may lie awake trying to solve problems or stressing about what happened. This is a very individual issue. Pay attention to your thought patterns and how you want to feel, and then choose a type of journaling that leaves you calm and comfortable, not overthinking. And, if journaling doesn't work for you or feed your soul, don't do it!

BODY CARE

My favorite part of my bedtime routine is self-care for my body. This is when I put on body lotion, giving my skin some moisturizer for those sun exposed areas. I love to put on a little face and eye cream so my face is extra moisturized and can heal and regenerate during the night.

If my body is sore, I put on arnica or hemp salve and give the sore areas a little massage. This is a true sleep aid, so I don't wake up due to aching muscles. It's also a great time to give gratitude for your body.

If you use any kind of light therapy for your skin or teeth, use it early in your bedtime routine so the light doesn't stimulate your brain to become more alert.

HERBAL TEA

Sip on a cup of herbal tea, such as chamomile or valerian root tea, before bedtime to promote relaxation and prepare your body for sleep. Avoid caffeinated beverages, as they can interfere with your ability to fall asleep. You can turn on the water for the tea as the first step of your bedtime routine. Then you can have your warm and calming tea to take with you as you prepare yourself for sleep.

LISTENING TO CALMING MUSIC

Many people love to listen to music to create a soothing atmosphere before bed. Choose music with a slow tempo and minimal lyrics to promote relaxation and ease your mind into a restful state. Some people prefer sounds of nature: waves, wind, or birds to soothe them into the night. Become aware of what is soothing for you, what you love to listen to, and what gives you the most peace. And, it might be silence!

Make sure the device has a shut off mechanism, so the music or sound doesn't continue all night. Also become aware if it wakes you up when it turns off. If this is the case, you may want to use it only as you are preparing to go to sleep.

CANDLE LIGHT

Lighting a candle in the bedroom can signal to the brain that it's time to sleep. For many, it creates a peaceful and intimate space that signals the drawing in of energy to your body so you can heal and rejuvenate during sleep. If using a scented candle, be aware of what affects that scent has on you both emotionally and physically. Some scents are very pleasant for us when we smell them but could be irritating and cause congestion if used over a longer period of time. Many people prefer unscented candles for this reason. Make sure to blow out the candle before you close your eyes!

GENTLE STRETCHING

So often our body becomes tight during the day, perhaps because we're sitting a lot, or holding our body in a certain position, and even when we've exercised and used our muscles to the point of soreness. Incorporate gentle stretching or yoga poses into your bedtime routine to release physical tension and promote relaxation. Become aware of where the pain, tightness, or congestion lives in your body. Is it in your neck, shoulders, or back? Focus on stretches or yoga poses that release that tension, using your breath to aid that release.

We'll go into more techniques to physically relax your body in the chapter, "Sleep Hack #4: Body Relaxation Techniques."

SAYING "GOODNIGHT" TO WORRIES AND THOUGHTS

As part of your bedtime routine, practice saying "goodnight" to your worries and thoughts. Acknowledge any concerns or anxieties you may have, and then consciously choose to set them aside as you prepare for sleep. You can also journal about these worries and thoughts, putting them down physically as well as mentally. And, if you wake up later thinking about them, you can consciously put them aside again. This practice helps ease your mind and prevents rumination, allowing you to drift off to sleep more easily.

AROMATHERAPY

Aromatherapy can soothe the mind, body, and spirit as part of a tranquil bedtime ritual. Aromatic essential oils have been used for centuries to promote relaxation, reduce stress, and improve sleep quality.

According to a study on hospitalized heart patients, aromatherapy reduced anxiety, increased sleep, and stabilized the blood pressure of patients. Research suggests that inhaling the aroma of essential oils can stimulate the limbic system in the brain, which is involved in emotions, memory, and arousal. This can lead to a cascade of physiological responses, including relaxation and stress reduction, making essential oils an effective tool for improving sleep quality.[2]

DIFFUSING ESSENTIAL OILS

Invest in a high-quality essential oil diffuser to disperse aromatic essential oils into the air in your bedroom. Choose calming essential oils such as lavender, chamomile, or bergamot to promote relaxation and prepare your body for sleep. Bergamot essential oil is known for its citrusy and uplifting aroma, which can help reduce stress and anxiety, promoting relaxation and restful sleep. Diffuse essential oils for 30 minutes to an hour before bedtime to create a soothing atmosphere.

2. Cho, M., Min, E., Hur, M., & Lee, M. "Effects of Aromatherapy on the Anxiety, Vital Signs, and Sleep Quality" Evidence Based Complementary Alternative Med. (2013) 2013: 381381. www.ncbi.nlm.nih.gov/pmc/articles/PMC3588400/

TOPICAL APPLICATION

Create a DIY essential oil sleep blend by diluting a few drops of your favorite essential oils with a carrier oil such as fractionated coconut oil or almond oil. Massage the blend into your temples, wrists, or the soles of your feet before bedtime to promote relaxation and improve sleep quality. Be sure to perform a patch test before applying essential oils to your skin to check for any adverse reactions.

We love lavender oil on the soles of our feet before bed. Lavender essential oil is one of the most popular and widely studied essential oils for promoting relaxation and improving sleep quality. Its calming aroma has been shown to reduce anxiety and stress, leading to improved sleep duration and quality.[3]

BEDTIME BATH

Add a few drops of essential oils to a warm bath before bedtime to create a luxurious and relaxing experience. Choose calming essential oils such as lavender, chamomile, or sandalwood to soothe your senses and prepare your body for sleep. Chamomile essential oil is a great choice since it promotes relaxation and improves sleep quality. It contains compounds that have sedative properties, making it an ideal choice for promoting restful sleep. Enjoy a leisurely soak in an aromatic bath to unwind and promote relaxation before bedtime.

LET YOUR BEDTIME ROUTINE LURE YOU IN

Having a relaxing bedtime routine is one of the most fun parts of going to sleep! Going into the bedroom when you're getting ready to go to sleep, lighting a candle, putting on music, drawing the shades,

---

3. Cho, M., Min, E., Hur, M., & Lee, M. "Effects of Aromatherapy on the Anxiety, Vital Signs, and Sleep Quality" Evidence Based Complementary Alternative Med. (2013) 2013: 381381. www.ncbi.nlm.nih.gov/pmc/articles/PMC3588400/

turning off the overhead lights all start the process of your nighttime sleep ritual.

This is about having time that's all for you, for your health, and your well-being. You can actually feel your brain and body starting to relax when you take the time to establish this habit of slowing down and nurturing yourself. You can create this nighttime oasis to give yourself the gift of a peaceful and restful sleep.

SLEEP HACK #3: LIMITING
SCREEN TIME BEFORE BED

The body relaxes as it feels the balm
of no more news feed, say goodnight to the phone,
Now you are in the sleeping zone.

IN THIS CHAPTER, we'll look at the effects of screen time on sleep quality and discuss strategies for limiting exposure before bedtime. The use of electronic devices such as smartphones, tablets, and computers has become increasingly prevalent in today's society. It seems that there's not a time or place when they're not present and being used. In the timeline of human development, this is a new phenomenon, although there are certainly millions of people now on the planet who have had the experience of the ever-present phone throughout their lifetime.

With the advent of personal use electronic devices, we've brought EMFs (electromagnetic waves) into our daily exposure. Multiply that close connection of the phone to our ear (brain), daily computer use, and all the cell towers, boosters, and smart meters across our country, and we have a bombardment of EMFs that our bodies have never experienced before.

Everyone understands that EMFs can impact the human body,

although we as a society, or in our body of science, do not fully realize what the influence is or will be. Some people are more susceptible to its negative effects than others. The blue light from cell phones and screens are the visual component of EMFs.

Let's explore the impact of screen time on the brain and sleep and learn how to establish healthy digital habits so we can get to sleep faster and stay asleep longer.

BLUE LIGHT AND ITS EFFECT ON SLEEP

Blue light is a type of light emitted by electronic devices such as smartphones, tablets, and computers. A study published in the Proceedings of the National Academy of Sciences found that participants who used electronic devices before bed took longer to fall asleep, experienced less restorative sleep, and reported higher levels of daytime sleepiness compared to those who avoided screens before bed.[1]

Exposure to blue light, especially in the evening, can suppress the production of melatonin, a hormone that is produced in the pineal gland in the brain and regulates sleep-wake cycles - our circadian rhythms. Melatonin tells our brain and body that it's time to go to sleep, and it is released in response to darkness. In other words, if there isn't any darkness (because you're looking at the blue light of your screen), your pineal gland won't release melatonin, and you won't get sleepy.

We all want to get better sleep, but why is it so hard to put down the darn phone?

Many of us have developed habits around catching up with our news feed, our favorite music, podcast, movie, or tv show before bed. But if we want better sleep, it's best to shift our screen time activities to earlier in the day or evening, so that we can get the most of our

---

1. Chang, A., Aeschbach, D., Duffy, F., & Czeisler, C. "Evening use of light-emitting eReaders negatively affects sleep, circadian timing, and next-morning alertness" Proceedings of the National Academy of Sciences. (2014) 112 (4) 1232-1237

sleeping hours. Establishing a digital curfew is one way to put a stop to excessive screen time before bed.

DIGITAL CURFEW

Think of a digital curfew as your personal boundary to reinforce your self-care. Wouldn't it feel great to wake up refreshed and inspired to have a great day? Having the intention to shut off devices when you start getting ready for bed will help you get to sleep faster and easier.

Set a specific time each evening (at least 30 minutes before lights out) to power down your electronic devices and engage in relaxing activities. Add a digital curfew to your bedtime routine that you created in, "Sleep Hack #2: Establishing a Relaxing Bedtime Routine."

About 30 minutes before you plan to go to bed might also be the time when you start turning the lights in your home down or off. It's time to put the devices to bed so they can get charged up too! Leaving the device charging unit in a different room can alleviate the temptation to pick it up again, as well as keep the EMFs out of your bedroom.

Some people make the bed off limits for digital devices and remove electronic devices from the bedside table at night. If you do have your device in the bedroom, make sure to turn off notifications and your ringer (unless necessary).

This digital curfew, of course, includes the television. While many people use TV to wind down from the day, leaving the tv on as a sleep aid can be extremely counterproductive. Volume changes from commercial breaks, scary music, and other distractions can wake you up, create fear or panic, and largely disrupt your ability to fall asleep and stay asleep. The best solution is to turn the tv off at least an hour before bed. Many people don't have a tv in their bedroom at all!

BREAKING THE HABIT

Recognize when you're using screens out of habit rather than necessity. Ask yourself if looking at your phone is what you really want to be doing. Is there something more meaningful or relaxing that you'd rather do?

Make a conscious effort to replace screen time with activities that fill you up: perhaps that's a conversation with a partner or a much needed self-care treat. There are many ideas for this in the preceding chapter, "Sleep Hack #2: Establishing a Relaxing Bedtime Routine."

Breaking the habit of using electronic devices before bed can be challenging, but in the long run, it will profoundly impact your health and happiness. You get to have restful sleep and a healthy sleep-wake cycle!

WHAT YOU CAN CREATE

By understanding the impact of screen time on sleep quality and implementing strategies to reduce screen time before bed, you can create a more conducive environment for falling asleep and staying asleep throughout the night. Establishing a digital curfew will signal to your brain that it's time to unwind and prepare for a restful night's sleep.

SLEEP HACK #4: BODY RELAXATION AND ENERGETIC RELEASE TECHNIQUES

Good night, toes, all the way to our nose

IN THIS SLEEP HACK, we'll examine relaxation techniques that can help alleviate tension, calm the mind, and promote restful sleep. These techniques are best done **in bed** because you may fall asleep immediately! From progressive muscle relaxation and visualizations to methods using the energetic systems of the body, let's investigate which relaxing process will create your optimal conditions for falling asleep, staying asleep, and getting back to sleep.

PROGRESSIVE MUSCLE RELAXATION

Progressive muscle relaxation (PMR) is a relaxation technique that involves systematically tensing and relaxing different muscle groups in the body. Start by tensing and then relaxing each muscle group in your body, starting from your toes and working your way up to your head. By progressively relaxing each muscle group, you can release physical tension and promote relaxation throughout your entire body. Research has shown that PMR can reduce muscle tension, alleviate stress, and improve sleep quality.[1] Make sure to breathe during this technique, as holding your breath as you tense can be counterproductive.

RELAXATION VISUALIZATION

For a less dynamic relaxation technique, but one that's still very helpful, visualize your body relaxing starting at your toes. Move through your toes, your feet, your ankles, the calves of your legs, your knees, and up your body with that level of specificity. You can wiggle the area to start the relaxation as you visualize the muscles themselves smoothing, relaxing, and turning into butter!

We store so much tension in our body. Everyone has their own unique places where their muscles stay tight longer. Where do you have that extra tightness or tension? Give that area a little love in this visualization.

Make sure to breathe during this process. And don't forget to relax the neck and jaw, all around your eyes and forehead and the back of the head. When we're thinking during the day, we create a lot of tension in those areas around our brain. Even if we only did this visualization on the head, we would signal to the brain that it's time to sleep! It's time to relax all that thinking and say good night.

And, just for those brain geeks out there, relaxing and saying good night to the various areas of the brain is very helpful too! Good night, visual cortex, while I close my eyes to sleep. Good night, hypothalamus, you can put sleep on auto pilot. Good night, hippocampus, I don't need to remember a thing. Good night, Amygdala, I have nothing to fear!

---

1. Nunez, K., "The benefits of progressive muscle relaxation and how to do it" Healthline.com. 2020 www.healthline.com/health/progressive-muscle-relaxation

BRINGING YOUR ENERGY BACK TO YOURSELF WITH CORETALK™ HOLISTIC HEALING

Many times a day we may be sending energy out from our body (our auric field) to another person, place, or thing in order to obtain a certain outcome. In other words, we might send our energy out to another person to help them think a certain way, make a decision, or to do something. Often when we send this energy out, we don't get it back. As time goes on, we may leave a lot of our energy out of our own auric field, and we can become energetically depleted and physically exhausted.

It's very important to bring our energy back so we can use it to manifest our own unique gifts and vision. When we do this as a nightly practice, we're practicing good energetic hygiene and keeping our energy for our own selves, where we really need it!

Process to bring your energy back into yourself.

1. Put your hands out in front of you, palms facing out.
2. Make the intention to gather all your energy back from wherever it is, across time and place.
3. Visualize your energy coming back into your hands. (Some people will feel a buzzing or a fullness there.)
4. Usher your energy into your body with your hands in a gathering motion.
5. Bring your hands to your heart, your solar plexus, your belly, your throat, all of your chakras, or wherever you feel called to place your hands.
6. Breathe in your energy to the entirety of your body.
7. Continue to gather and bring your energy into your body until you feel complete.
8. You may give yourself a hug to pat all your energy into your body.

RUNNING MERIDIANS WITH CORETALK™ HOLISTIC HEALING

One of the bedtime relaxation techniques that we love to do is run our energetic body meridians. Body meridians influence different body systems, organs, muscles as well as carry emotions. For instance, the bladder meridian influences the bladder, the urinary system, your spinal muscles and the emotion of fear. Many people have a lot of fear running in their lives, so we love to run our bladder meridian before we go to sleep or if we wake up in the middle of the night with fearful, anxious, or worried thoughts.

Running your bladder meridian is simple. Using two hands, put your pointer fingers between your eyebrows on your forehead and run them in a straight line over your head, down your back and all the way down the back of your legs to your little toes. Then put your hands in the arch of your feet and run them up the inside of your legs and up the middle of your torso where a sweater zipper would be and up to your collar bones. While doing this, take a breath and say, I release all the fear around this situation.

You may feel immediate release and the sensation of lightness, or it may take a few minutes to feel this, or you may feel nothing. However, if you run this meridian when you feel fear, you'll experience a lifting of the fear and an ability to look at the situation differently. On the other side of fear is courage, and we all want to have courage to do the things we want to do.

MEDITATION

We also recommend that meditation be part of your bedtime or nighttime routine to fall asleep or get back to sleep quickly and easily. We've devoted the next chapter, Sleep Hack #5: Using Meditation to Fall Asleep," to this technique as it is a very important factor for your quality of sleep, and for the overall quality of your life.

EXPLORE THE POSSIBILITIES

There are many other body and mind relaxation techniques out there. When you find one that works for you, use it until it doesn't! Then try something else. As we become more aware of our own sleep issues and solutions, we grow and change and use sleep as a way of healing all areas of our lives. This is part of being an amazing human! Because we need to spend one third of our lives asleep, we can use that time to fully and consciously regenerate and heal our mind, body, and spirit.

SLEEP HACK #5: USING MEDITATION TO FALL ASLEEP

Good night, noise, good night, light,
good night, to anything that leads to a fight.

THE MOST IMPORTANT area of your sleep sanctuary is not just your bedroom, but in your brain! If it is occupied with stress and worry, it can be difficult to cultivate an effective sleep routine. This is where meditation comes in.

In this sleep hack, we'll explore how meditation can help calm a busy mind, reduce stress, and promote relaxation, all while setting the stage for deep restorative sleep. We'll look at different ways of meditating so you can find one that works best for you.

Creating a regular meditation practice outside of your sleep routine can be helpful, but for this sleep hack, we'll look at how to use meditation as a part of your sleep routine when you want to fall asleep. We suggest that you meditate in bed when you want to fall asleep or get back to sleep. You could meditate before getting into bed, but by meditating in bed, you can use the meditation to take you directly into sleep. We like to think of it as **Beditation**.

BENEFITS OF MEDITATION FOR SLEEP

Meditation has many benefits for sleep quality and overall well-being. Meditation is especially useful to calm and focus the mind on what we want to think about, not on the worries or fears that our mind often focuses on.

What we know from working with clients, specifically around improving their sleep, is that if you don't give the mind something to focus on, it will focus on what it thinks you need to pay attention to. Picture this: you're lying in bed, and your mind is racing with thoughts about tomorrow's to-do list or that embarrassing thing you said five years ago. Sound familiar?

Racing or worried thoughts will often lead to feelings of anxiety and emotional distress. Meditation gives you a way to say, "I'm not going there" when your brain wants to take you down an emotional rabbit hole.

WHAT IS MEDITATION?

Now, let's break down what meditation is all about. Think of it as a daily mental workout for your brain, where you carve out some time to focus your mind on a specific object, thought, or activity. Whether it's focusing on your breath, repeating a calming mantra, or simply observing your thoughts without judgment, the goal is to train your mind to find stillness and clarity amidst the chaos of daily life. By making meditation a regular part of your routine, you're essentially giving your mind the tools it needs to stay focused, redirect unhelpful thoughts, and cultivate a sense of inner peace and calm. It's like hitting the reset button for your brain, helping you unwind and recharge after a long day.

MEDITATION: ANCIENT WISDOM, MODERN BENEFITS

People have been practicing meditation for thousands of years, with some of the earliest records dating back to ancient India and China.

Fast forward to today, and meditation is more popular than ever, thanks to its wide array of health benefits, making meditation a one-stop shop for overall well-being. It's been shown to increase happiness, decrease depression and anxiety, and even improve memory and focus. So, whether you're a seasoned meditator or a curious newcomer, there's no denying the powerful impact that meditation can have on your mind, body, and sleep quality.[1]

WHEN SHOULD I MEDITATE?

In addition to using meditation at bedtime, we recommend meditating first thing in the morning for 20 minutes. To put this into practice we used the acronym RPM (Rise, Pee, Meditate) to make it our morning ritual. This has been our daily practice for many years. Ideally, we also like to meditate right after work (RAW), but this can sometimes be a little more challenging when your day is moving along.

Having a dedicated meditation practice outside of your sleep routine can significantly enhance the effectiveness of your bedtime meditation. The more you meditate, the better equipped you become at calming both your mind and body, which at bedtime leads to falling asleep more easily.

In clinical research, meditation has emerged as a powerful tool for enhancing mental well-being, particularly in combating stress.[2] Since stress often manifests as insomnia, characterized by difficulty falling and staying asleep, integrating meditation into your routine can effectively promote relaxation and alleviate stress-related sleep disturbances, especially when practiced at bedtime.

Let's look at different types of meditation so you can experiment and see which ones are the most relaxing for you. We find that many

1. Rusch HL, Rosario M, Levison LM, et al. "The effect of mindfulness meditation on sleep quality: a systematic review and meta-analysis of randomized controlled trials" Annals of the New York Academy of Sciences. (2019) 1445(1):5-16. https://pubmed. ncbi.nlm.nih.gov/30575050/
2. Mayo Clinic. (2024) "A Fast, Simple Way to Reduce Stress"

of the following types of meditations can be used together as part of your sleep routine. We'll describe what some of those combinations look like and how to use them in a way that flows and leads you into a restful sleep.

MINDFULNESS MEDITATION

Mindfulness meditation involves focusing your attention on the present moment without judgment, allowing you to cultivate awareness and acceptance of your thoughts and feelings. It can be an effective way to alleviate recurring stress from situations that develop at work and in relationships.

As we go through different types of meditation and how to use them to fall asleep, you'll realize that using mindfulness meditation to be in the moment is an essential part of any meditation you use as part of your sleep routine.

BODY SCAN MEDITATION

Body scan meditation is all about bringing awareness to areas of your body that might be holding tension. Start by focusing your attention on your toes and moving upward, one part of your body at a time, until you get up to your head. Notice any areas of tension or discomfort and allow them to soften and relax as you pause and breathe deeply in those areas.

Body Scan Meditation is a great way to start your bedtime meditation routine because releasing tension in your body will allow you to begin to relax so you can fall asleep.

BREATH AWARENESS MEDITATION

Breath awareness meditation helps anchor your attention to the present moment so you can quiet your mind. As you settle into bed, focus on the sensation of your breath as it enters and leaves your body.

We suggest placing one hand on your stomach and the other on your chest. Notice the rise and fall of your abdomen with each breath, allowing yourself to become fully present and centered.

This is especially good for people who tend to hold their breath during the day. If you find yourself getting distracted and want to bring more awareness to the breath, you can introduce counting, four counts on the inhale and four counts on the exhale. This will bring your mind's focus back to your breath and into the present moment. Later we'll talk about using breath awareness with a mantra last in your meditation routine because it is really effective in inducing sleep!

LOVING-KINDNESS MEDITATION

There's nothing like giving yourself a little love to help dissolve the stress and frustration that can come with insomnia.

Loving-kindness meditation can cultivate feelings of compassion and well-being by shifting attention away from worry and concern. Close your eyes and silently repeat phrases such as "May I be safe; may I be happy, and may I be healthy." Extend these wishes to yourself and others to create a sense of connection and kindness that will promote relaxation and prepare you for sleep.

You can use Loving-Kindness Meditation as part of your sleep meditation routine whenever your mind kicks up the worry quotient. This is especially helpful if you find yourself thinking of things that you can't do anything about at the moment. It's a way to put your worries to sleep for the night by shifting those concerns about your-self, others, and the world, to a feeling of love and kindness, knowing that all will be well. By leaving our troubles behind for the moment and cultivating that loving kindness for ourselves and others, we can drift off to sleep more quickly and easily.

In our healing work, CoreTalk™, when we have a loving-kindness conversation with our body, we put our hands on our heart and bring loving energy into our heart chakra. We repeat the words, "I love you; I love you; I love you!" reminding our body and mind of all the love we are filled with and that we have for ourselves and flooding our beings with peace and equanimity. We love to use this meditation in the middle of the night to get back to sleep fast.

GUIDED IMAGERY AND VISUALIZATION

Guided imagery and visualization are relaxation techniques that involve creating mental images of peaceful and calming scenes. By immersing yourself in a vivid imaginary experience, you can distract your mind from intrusive thoughts and promote relaxation. Guided imagery and visualization can be practiced using audio recordings, guided meditation apps, or simply by visualizing calming scenes in your mind. Many people like to think of waves at the beach, or being in a redwood forest, or in a meadow. Whatever image soothes your brain and relaxes your body is perfect for you.

If you're using an app on your phone, make sure to change the brightness settings to low or "nighttime" so that you're not getting bright light from your screen.

MANTRA MEDITATION

A mantra can be anything that you repeat over and over again in your mind. It can be a prayer, an affirmation, a favorite saying, or a loving thought. For example, some people choose a bible verse, or the Serenity prayer, or perhaps, even the affirmation, "I am loved," or "I have peaceful sleep." One of Greg's favorites is, "Sleep, Sleep," with each breath.

Or, if you realize you're anxious about something, you can create an affirmation that counters your anxiety. If you have a difficult project coming up at work, perhaps your affirmation is, "My project will be well received." Or if you're dealing with a difficult person, your affirmation could be "I have loving relationships in my life."

Or perhaps you think of gratitude instead of your troubles with, "I am grateful for what I have in my life."

WHAT MIGHT YOUR MANTRA BE?

On a lighter note, people have been counting sheep for millennia, and that is a mantra that indeed distracts the brain with the monotony necessary to relax and sleep.

As with any meditation, if your mind begins to wander, you can bring it back to the meditation again with the mantra or focusing on your breath; no judgment, no worries.

You might be thinking, "What mantra is going to work best for me?"

Everyone is different, especially when it comes to what your mind focuses on. Start with something simple. We suggest using a simple mantra meditation like thinking the word 'sleep' with each breath in and each breath out. If that works for you, keep doing it. If after 5 nights you find your mind still wandering relentlessly, try a different meditation technique.

WHAT YOU'LL GET

All of these meditation techniques incorporate mindfulness as a way of being in the moment and calming your mind. By using one or more of these meditation techniques, you'll be able to create a calm place in your mind which will lower your stress level and make it easier for you to fall asleep. It's as easy as paying attention to your breath.

You can begin to meditate as you go through your bedtime routine in preparation for getting into bed. You can use a visual meditation right after you turn off the light to relax and then move on to a mantra meditation to focus on sleep. You can meditate on love or gratitude in the middle of the night to move the mind away from stressors so you can get back to sleep. Feel into which technique best suits the issue you're having so you can get back to sleep quickly and easily.

When you incorporate your meditative vibe into your entire sleep routine, you'll cultivate a sense of peace and relaxation that sets the stage for a restful night's sleep.

SLEEP HACK #6: HOW CONSCIOUS BREATHING GETS YOU INTO THE SLEEP GROOVE

Our breathing brings closer what everyone knows,
That the lightness within is what brings us such peace
and gives us good sleep so our healing does increase.

So, what role does breathing play in helping us improve our sleep? Breathing, especially when you want to leave your worries behind and get your body and brain to relax, is the most important component to good sleep.

We're going to look at a specific type of breathing called conscious breathing. And we're going to use conscious breathing to anchor the other sleep hacks into your sleep routine.

It's important to become aware of how you breathe now and what your breathing patterns are. Once you have that understanding, you can make conscious choices about how to use your breath as you internalize the other sleep hacks into your body. Then, you'll quickly begin to get results without having to think about the sleep hacks. You'll literally breathe them into your sleep routine.

WHAT IS CONSCIOUS BREATHING?

So, what is conscious breathing and how does it affect our health and wellness in regard to sleep? Very simply, conscious breathing is awareness and observation of the components of breathing: the inhalation, length of breath, fullness of lungs and the speed and volume of the exhalation.

But, before getting deeper into what conscious breathing is and why we might want to use it, let's take a simple breath. Take a relaxed, easy breath in, paying attention to the air coming in and the lungs beginning to fill, and when you feel like you want to exhale, let your breath go back out. You have just taken a conscious breath. How was it?

Basically, you paid attention to your breath. You watched yourself take a breath and guided the steps from the beginning to the end of one breath. Conscious breathing is doing this over and over again until your body breathes the way you want it to instead of the reactive way you breathe habitually when you're not consciously thinking about breathing.

When we want to fall asleep, we can use conscious breathing to integrate all the other sleep hacks you're learning. It becomes the glue, or really the thread, that brings them into balance as you integrate the sleep hacks into the pattern of your sleep routine.

WHY USE CONSCIOUS BREATHING?

But why would you want to breathe consciously? Your body will breathe automatically, even forcing you to inhale if too much CO_2 (carbon dioxide) builds up in the blood going through the lungs. Breathing *consciously* allows us to use the breath as a tool to calm anxiety, stress, and pain IN THE MOMENT. One of the powerful results of conscious breathing is that it is an anchor to BEING in the moment.

And when it comes to going to sleep and getting back to sleep, being in the moment is one of the keys to a successful sleep mindset.

Our brains' habitual thinking tends to throw us out of the present moment and into the past or future. Under our brains' control, we tend to hold our breath when anxious or when stressful memories come up. And in extreme situations, it's hard to catch our breath while having a panic attack. And, if that panic attack is showing up in the middle of the night, it's nearly impossible to get back to sleep quickly.

THE POWER OF BEING IN THE MOMENT

Knowing how the brain tends to go off on tangents, we can use conscious breathing to reign it in and even purposefully use it to let go of stressful thoughts and feelings. In other words, when the brain goes into overdrive, we can use our breath to stay in the moment and see that things are not as bad as the brain may be portraying them. Then we can refocus our active brain to what we really want: to go to sleep or go back to sleep. When we use our breath to create a calm mindset for sleep, that mindset will make it easier to stay asleep too.

With all this detail about breathing you might be thinking, how am I going to get good at this stuff? Through millennia, life coaches, yogis, spiritual leaders, masters and teachers of martial and fine arts, have taught about the importance of using breath to improve the outcome of life and whatever task is at hand in the moment. But the question is, where do we start? What level of expertise is needed, and how do we know we're breathing in a way that's going to help us get better sleep?

YOU CAN DO THIS!

This is where it gets good. We don't have to learn more or do more to take advantage of what the breath has to offer. It's simply about letting go of the things our brain has made up that have burdened the breath and made it less than easy and natural. And, letting go happens by watching our breath, especially if our brain starts to go off into negative territory when we want to be going to sleep. In essence, we are minding our brain by consciously watching our breath. As we pay attention to our breath, we begin to see when the brain starts to inter-ject its potentially chaotic rendering of the moment, and, instead of allowing the brain to portray chaos, we breathe and choose calm.

As a consequence of simply taking the breath in and letting it go out in a relaxed manner, we are training our autonomic nervous system to help us be more relaxed. This leads to a healthier, more balanced way to go through our day and bring that calm relaxed feeling into our bedtime routine.

Over time, a conscious breathing practice begins to be part of our everyday breathing routine. We can dip in and out of conscious breathing, feeling more balanced in the moment without having to consciously manage each breath. Conscious breathing will become an effortless feeling that you can easily bring into your sleep routine to go to sleep, get back to sleep, and stay asleep.

USING CONSCIOUS BREATHING TO ANCHOR THE SLEEP HACKS

There's another powerful and practical side to conscious breathing that can affect everything we do, especially as we integrate the sleep hacks into our bedtime routine.

Each night as you begin your new bedtime routine, consciously use your breath with each of the sleep hacks as you go through them. Stretching can be more relaxed with the breath; turning the lights down becomes a meditation; reading is relaxed and without any goal in mind; preparing the bath or putting essential oils in a diffuser, all become an act of relaxation and letting go as you breath away any stress from the day and allow your routine and your breath to guide you into your sleepy time.

There is no special method to conscious breathing. No counting, no holding the breath for a certain number of counts, no special exhale sound or mindset. It is simply taking one breath at a time, allowing yourself to be consciously aware of the breath going in and out of your body as you fall asleep.

WITH EACH BREATH

Now that you have all the info you need to bring conscious breathing into your sleep routine, you'll be able to add the simple meditation mantra that you created in the previous chapter. As you repeat the mantra in your mind, your awareness of your breath through conscious breathing will anchor your ability to calm your mind and fall asleep.

Your sleep mantra can be repeated in the rhythm of each breath you take or repeated over and over as you breath, without any specific connection to your breath, other than awareness. If your mind begins to wander, use the breath as a reminder to bring you back to the mantra.

Keep it simple and be kind to yourself if your mind gets busy. It's all about progress, not perfection, when it comes to creating awareness with the breath and using a mantra to help your mind relax.

KEEP IT SIMPLE

Breathing is natural and something we don't really have to think about. But, we can use our breath to consciously create more awareness of how we feel, mentally and physically, in the moment. When we use that awareness as part of our bedtime routine, and ultimately as the final step to actually falling asleep, this special time, our sleep time, is enhanced in a way that can give us insight into how we can use the breath to improve all areas of our life.

SLEEP HACK #7: CULTIVATING A POSITIVE SLEEP MINDSET

Good night, brain, good night, thinking train.
Good night and sleep tight, while asleep we remain.

IN THIS SLEEP HACK, we'll delve into the importance of cultivating a positive sleep mindset. Your emotions, thoughts, and beliefs about sleep can significantly influence your ability to fall asleep and stay asleep throughout the night. By shifting your perspective on sleep from one of worry and frustration to one of relaxation and trust, you can create a more conducive environment for a long and restful sleep, night after night. Creating a Sleep Intention is a powerful, but simple technique to help you shift into knowing that you can have restful, calm, and restorative sleep every night, no matter what the circumstances.

Most people agree that having a positive mindset attracts more positivity in life. The Law of Attraction exemplifies this - whatever you think about attracts similar energy. If you think negatively, you'll attract or multiply negative thoughts or energy; if you think positively, you'll attract positive thoughts or energy.

Thinking positively is especially important for sleep because we are highly affected by our emotions, thoughts, and beliefs. If we're upset, angry, worried, or anxious (long term or in the moment), we can easily disrupt our night's sleep.

One of the biggest tools in our sleep tool chest is our control over how we think about sleep, not just at bedtime, but all the time! And, because we may have had many years of non-optimal sleep habits, it can take time to reverse these patterns so that we can consistently have the beautiful sleep that we so crave night after night.

It's very natural to develop negative thought patterns around sleep when there may have been difficult experiences, memories, and emotions that have played out at night or in bed. We get into how to heal some of these very important issues in the next chapter, "What If It's More Serious?"

In this Sleep Hack, we're going to establish a Sleep Intention, which is a positive outlook on sleep overall. You'll be able to refer to this positive intention at any time - day or night - to reinforce to your brain how you want it to be. This will help your brain change its neural pathways to the outlook and belief that you want, not just the way it has been. You can do this. You don't have to live within the confines of the old memories, hurts, and negative emotions from the past. You can create the life you want, starting right now.

And, because the brain requires a little time to reprogram itself (with you helping it), we'll start this process right away, and you can begin to work your sleep magic! We'll give ourselves the benefit of positive thoughts and beliefs when it comes to sleep, so we can feel confident in our ability to fall asleep and stay asleep. We'll shift our habits and patterns away from those old negative neural pathways into more neutral and even positive belief patterns that can start right now.

CREATING A SLEEP INTENTION

Setting a Sleep Intention is important so that you clearly define how you want your sleep to be. In doing so, you're telling yourself and the universe what you desire. And remember, you get to have what you want! With focus and intention, you can make this incredible piece of self-care become a beautiful reality for you.

Remember, in the second chapter, how we looked at our sleep patterns, issues, and beliefs? You identified the first issue you wanted to work on and have been using the Sleep Hacks to deal with that issue. You also started listing your emotional settings and beliefs around sleep. You have, probably by now, identified several (or many) beliefs that you may have around sleep.

Now, we'll create a sleep intention that speaks to your most detrimental sleep belief. This is especially important so you can put all of your energy toward the same goal, giving your brain a job to carry out your wishes about sleep. And, remember, this could take some time to become your reality, so be patient and remember that your brain and your body are working in the background to make this happen for you.

Here are some examples of Sleep Intentions:

- Sleep comes easily to me
- I have peaceful sleep every night
- I fall asleep quickly and easily
- I go to bed early so I can get the sleep I need
- I sleep through the night
- I sleep 7 to 8 hours most nights
- I sleep well regardless of what happened during the day
- I love going to bed
- I am safe when I sleep
- Sleep is a restorative and healing time for me
- I fall back to sleep easily
- My bedroom is my sleep sanctuary
- I trust my body to fall asleep naturally
- I am relaxed and ready for a restful night's sleep

PICK YOUR SLEEP INTENTION

When you pick your sleep intention, you can shift your internal beliefs about sleep. You can repeat it during the day when negative thoughts or beliefs come up around how you're going to sleep. The intention will counter any negative beliefs about sleep and take the focus off negative sleep experiences from the past. The more positive energy you put toward your sleep, the more rejuvenating and deeper your sleep will be.

You'll have to reinforce this intention, and it may not work every time, but when you set your body, mind, and spirit to something, you can achieve it. We love to write our sleep intentions on several sticky notes and post one in the bathroom, one by the bed, and one on the computer or on the refrigerator - wherever you'll see them often.

Sleep intentions are meant to shift and change over time as you achieve better and longer sleep. Make sure to always have a sleep intention, but allow it to change as you change.

INCORPORATING POSITIVE SLEEP INTENTIONS

A sleep intention can also be a sleep affirmation. Incorporating positive sleep affirmations into your bedtime routine can help calm your mind and signal to your brain that it's time to unwind and prepare for sleep.

You can also use visualization and guided imagery techniques with your sleep affirmations, mentally picturing yourself in a peaceful and serene sleep environment. By visualizing yourself drifting off to sleep peacefully and waking up feeling refreshed and rejuvenated, you can create a positive mental image of sleep and reinforce positive associations with bedtime.

WHAT YOU'LL GET

Cultivating a positive sleep mindset is essential for overcoming insomnia and improving sleep quality. By shifting your perspective on sleep, creating a sleep intention, and incorporating it into your life, you can create a more supportive mental environment for restful sleep. Embrace a positive outlook on sleep, trust in your body's ability to rest and rejuvenate during the night, and you are setting the stage for a restful night's sleep and improved overall well-being.

AVOIDING SLEEP DISRUPTING ACTIVITIES

IN THIS CHAPTER, let's look at the various activities and behaviors that can disrupt your sleep-wake cycle and hinder your ability to fall asleep, go back to sleep, and stay asleep. From alcohol consumption and engaging in arguments to excessive exercise and late-night eating, we'll discuss the impact of these activities on sleep quality and provide tips for avoiding them before bedtime. By understanding the effects of these sleep-disrupting activities and establishing healthier pre-sleep routines (see Sleep Hack #2 and #3), you can create a more conducive environment for restful sleep.

CAFFEINE CONSUMPTION

Most people know that drinking coffee, tea, or soda with caffeine can keep you awake. However, caffeine affects people differently. Some people can drink it all day and still go to sleep and sleep all night. Other people can only have one or two servings before they're bouncing off the walls! How does caffeine affect you? If you want to improve your sleep and love your cup of Joe, experiment with timing and quantity. We found that we can't drink caffeine after 12:00 noon or our sleep will be affected. If you suspect caffeine is affecting your sleep, stop drinking anything with caffeine 4 to 6 (or more) hours before bedtime.

Many people have sworn off caffeine altogether because of its effects of hyping up the nervous system which makes them feel jumpy or agitated. Some people take time off drinking coffee and switch to green tea (which has comparable amounts of caffeine, but more antioxidants). Some people get stomach issues from coffee because non-organic coffee is heavily sprayed and grown with pesticides. When they switch to organic coffee, their stomach issues go away. You get to choose how you want to feel, not just at bedtime, but all day!

Another tip is to beware of hidden caffeine in soda, chocolate, and tea, as well as in pain relievers, weight loss pills, diuretics, and cold medicines. Read the label and check it out! These different sources of caffeine can add up over the course of the day. You may be getting more caffeine than you thought.

ALCOHOL CONSUMPTION

Alcohol has been used as a recreational drug and sleep aid for thousands of years. Some people have used it to manage their insomnia in order to relax and to go to sleep faster and easier. However, alcohol has been proven to be addictive, so drinking small amounts can often grow into larger amounts as the person develops a tolerance. Scientific research has shown that even small amounts of alcohol can be disruptive to sleep.[1]

While having a drink in the evening or before bed may initially create a relaxed and drowsy feeling, it creates a cascade of physiological events in your body that ultimately interferes with the quality of sleep in many ways. Here's a list of some of the effects:

---

1. Colrain, I., Nicholas, C., & Baker, F. "Alcohol and the Sleeping Brain" Handbook of Clinical Neurology (2014) 125: 415–431. www.ncbi.nlm.nih.gov/pmc/articles/PMC5821259

- Disrupts all stages of sleep, but especially REM sleep so you don't achieve deep, restorative sleep. Because of not entering deep sleep, you may have more vivid dreams or nightmares.
- Acts as a vasodilator that can increase heart rate causing discomfort and agitation and the likelihood of awakenings during the night. This vasodilation can also cause night sweats.
- Increases risk of obstructive sleep apnea (a potentially serious sleep disorder in which breathing repeatedly stops and starts) because it relaxes throat muscles.[2]
- Causes you to wake up in the middle of the night to go to the bathroom because it is a diuretic. Drinking alcohol is also very dehydrating which can cause a hangover in combination with sleep deprivation.

For a longer and more peaceful sleep, the best advice is to drink less than 2 drinks or glasses of wine and have a glass of water for each one. For best sleep, don't drink at all or stop drinking 4-6 hours before bedtime.

By the way, if you smoke, that may be wrecking your sleep as well, because nicotine is a stimulant and will keep you awake.

LATE-NIGHT EATING

Another thing we have to watch out for before bed is eating! Everyone has to eat, right? But sometimes what we eat and when we eat it can disrupt our sleep. Eating a heavy or spicy meal too close to bedtime makes for uncomfortable sleep because it activates your digestion leading to nighttime trips to the bathroom. Sleep usually slows down your digestive system so sometimes that heavy meal can sit like a

---

2. Simou, E., Britton, J., & Leonardi-Bee, J. "Alcohol and the risk of sleep apnoea: a systematic review and meta-analysis" Sleep medicine, (2018) 42, 38–46. www.ncbi.nlm.nih.gov/pmc/articles/PMC5840512/

lump in your stomach, and you're unable to get your ZZZs. Stop eating high-fat, high protein, and spicy foods at least 4 hours before bedtime.

If you're hungry, opt for a small piece of cheese and some sleep-friendly carbs, like crackers. But not too much!

EXCESSIVE EXERCISE

The only time exercising is an anti-sleep activity is if you do it right before bed. Overall, exercise is something you'll want to increase in your search for better sleep. Exercise is a sure way to feel better. It stimulates digestion, brain activity, and your lymphatic system. It lifts mood and reduces stress. It can strengthen circadian rhythms, promoting daytime alertness, and it can help bring on sleepiness at night.

Studies show that daytime physical activity may stimulate longer periods of slow-wave sleep, the deepest and most restorative stages of sleep. YAY!

However, engaging in vigorous exercise close to bedtime can be too stimulating. Exercise raises your body temperature and stimulates your nervous system, making it difficult to wind down and prepare for sleep. Aim to finish your workout a few hours before bedtime to allow your body time to cool down and relax.

ENGAGING IN STRESSFUL ACTIVITIES

Avoid engaging in stressful activities like arguments or heated discussions, conversations about money issues, or other negatively stimulating conversations before bedtime because they can elevate stress and anxiety levels, stimulating your mind and making it difficult to relax and fall asleep. Remember the phrase, "Never go to bed angry?" It's very hard to relax your brain and body when emotions and anxiety are high.

Many people turn off their phone to send a challenging (or triggering) call to voicemail after a certain time of night. Others avoid calling certain people at night knowing the conversation will be stressful. I make sure to do my bookkeeping before dinner, so I don't have to think about money at bedtime!

And, if you do happen to be stressed or angry before bed (it happens), remember Sleep Hacks #4-6, and run your body meridians to clear the anger and fear, do some mantra meditation, or some conscious breathing to relax yourself into a beautiful sleep.

WHAT YOU WILL GET

By avoiding sleep-disrupting activities, limiting caffeine and alcohol consumption, and avoiding arguments and stress, you are establishing your self-care healthy sleep routines! You are taking beautiful responsibility for how you feel every day and realizing that sleep is an important part of what allows you to feel vibrant, energetic and wholly YOU! You deserve long and restful sleep and the overall well-being that comes with it.

WHAT IF IT'S MORE SERIOUS?

IN OUR CLINICAL work at Self Health Institute, we see a lot of people with sleep issues, ranging from trauma related nightmares and night-time PTSD to COPD, acid reflux, sleep apnea, and chronic anxiety. All these issues, plus many other physical and mental conditions, affect the quality of our sleep and thus the quality of our lives. Since 1995, we've helped thousands of people regain healthy sleep habits and achieve long lasting sleep quality.

We believe that most chronic health and sleep issues are caused by adverse experiences combined with an unhealthy amount of toxins from pesticides, non-organic food, water additives, sugar, plastics, chemicals, and other inorganic substances. Add to that, any genetic predisposition to disease and inherited physical and mental negative emotional settings and beliefs, and you have a recipe for foundational sleep issues that, over time, disrupt your fundamental health and happiness in life.

Because of all these emotional and environmental challenges, we work with the body's internal energetic healing system, the chakras and meridians, to remove energetic and physical congestion and stagnation from the body's tissues - to literally get the issues out of the tissues. In this way, all the cells, organs, and body systems can naturally reset as they get an optimal flow of energy and nutrients.

ACES

In a landmark 1990's study conducted by Kaiser Permanente and the Center for Disease Control (CDC) in the U.S., adults were asked ten yes/no questions to determine the number of specific adverse experiences from their childhood through age 18. That study became known as the ACEs study. ACEs, or Adverse Childhood Experiences, are proven to have negative health effects across a lifetime.[1] These effects include, but are not limited to, heart attack, COPD, cancer, stroke, high blood pressure/hypertension and diabetes. Other effects include eating disorders, drug addiction, suicidal tendencies, and, as studies are now beginning to show, sleep disorders.

In the National Institute of Health, National Library of Medicine, an article entitled, *Adverse Childhood Experiences Are Associated With Adult Sleep Disorders: A Systematic Review,* details the correlation between ACEs and sleep disorders.[2] This systematic review showed "significant associations between sleep disorders including sleep apnea, narcolepsy, nightmare distress, sleep paralysis, and psychiatric sleep disorders with a history of childhood adversity."

These adverse childhood experiences can be related to/or caused by physical, sexual, or mental abuse, physical or emotional neglect, or household dysfunction including mental illness, drug abuse, maternal abuse, divorce, or incarceration.

The ACEs documented in the study are those that occur in childhood before the age of eighteen, and yet, adverse experiences can occur any time in life and still have detrimental effects on our ability to go to sleep, get back to sleep, and stay asleep. Living through diffi-

1. "About Adverse Childhood Experiences" Center for Disease Control" (2024) www.cdc.gov/aces/about/index.html

2. Kajeepeta, K., Gelaye, B., Jackson, C., and Williams, M., "Adverse childhood experiences are associated with adult sleep disorders: a systematic review" Sleep Medicine, (2015) Mar; 16(3): 320–330. www.ncbi.nlm.nih.gov/pmc/articles/PMC4635027/

cult experiences like natural disasters, a contentious divorce, any type of abuse, or death or separation from a loved one can cause trauma that results in the same types of devastating health conditions caused by ACEs.

Being an adult doesn't make us immune to the effects of difficult adverse experiences. Adult adverse experiences tend to trigger the actual neurological settings we developed from ACEs we had in childhood. And what's frustrating about adverse experiences we have as adults is that the strategies we use in the moment are many times a remake of what we developed as children to deal with the original or similar adverse experience.

And what we've found in working with adults since 1995 in our clinical CoreTalk™ Holistic Healing practice, is that in addition to chronic health issues, people who are affected by ACEs often suffer from high levels of self-doubt, procrastination, perfectionism, anxiety, and other negative emotional settings and behaviors that can cause negative outcomes in life, relationships, business, education, and wealth.

Do you know your ACEs score? To get more perspective on what and how many ACEs you had in your first 18 years, take the ACEs quiz here: www.acesquiz.com. It will give you a starting place to begin understanding this complex and highly studied metric and how it may be affecting your health and well-being now.

The tricky part about ACEs is that western allopathic medicine doesn't have a cure for it. Doctors can treat the symptoms of a disease caused by ACEs, but they have no clear path to curing the underlying core issues of ACEs.

SELF HEALTH INSTITUTE

This is where our work at Self Health Institute comes in. We have found that clinical use of our CoreTalk™ Holistic Healing therapy addresses and heals the effects of adverse childhood experiences. By working with the body's innate energetic healing system and following its powerful, yet simple set of instructions to initiate the healing process, over time we can heal the chronic health conditions that develop from adverse childhood experiences.

Because the chronic health challenges associated with ACEs are real and documented with significant empirical evidence and still not being addressed through allopathic medicine, we feel compelled to offer our insights and healing processes that have been developed over decades. The anecdotal evidence is clear. Our bodies know how to heal, and they know what has created the dis-ease. It's up to us to take the next steps.

CoreTalk™ Holistic Healing is not a substitute for consulting with your doctor. Consult a physician whenever you feel it is necessary. Energetic and naturopathic healing methods have been a mainstay of human health for millennia and continue to be at the forefront of our evolving human experience.

Understanding how our experiences, adverse or otherwise, affect our sleep is an integral part of solving any health issue, especially sleep issues that are at the core of our health at the deepest level. Remember that sleep time is healing time.

Importantly, other nighttime issues such as fear of the dark, night-mares, night sweats, and recurring phobias can be beautifully healed using your body's innate healing system.

If you would like to learn more about how to heal these issues, please contact us via email at support@selfhealthinstitute.com.

SLEEP ISSUE CASE STUDIES

Here are a few examples of how we've helped people get back to having rejuvenative and peaceful sleep. Many times, it's an easy fix for something that has been going on for decades. Other times, healing what is showing up as insomnia, involves taking a deeper look into how a person's life experiences have manifested as an inability to fall asleep or get restful sleep.

In the cases below, we used CoreTalk™ to talk with the client's body to help us discover the underlying issues causing lack of sleep. Many times sleep issues were accompanied by other physiological, emotional, mental, and energetic conditions that our client wanted to address.

To fully understand what we mean when we say "talk with your body" it may be helpful to watch this short video at www.selfhealthin stitute.com/coretalkdemo to see how we communicate with the body to tap into its healing wisdom. There, you'll see how we use Core-Talk™ to address whatever issue is showing up that needs attention. You'll see how we get answers to questions about health, relation-ships, wealth, and much more.

Imagine being able to do this type of healing for yourself. If you'd like to have more of an impact on your health outcomes, we can teach you how to heal your body using CoreTalk™. It's not difficult but takes some time to become accustomed to talking with your body about how you can affect your health. Using your body as the source of information about what is best for you and creating the confidence that you are strong and healthy and that your body heals perfectly is where you can start.

MY SLEEP JOURNEY

Before getting into case studies of our clients, I, (this is Greg speaking) want to talk about the ups and downs of my own sleep journey throughout my life. Hopefully, this will shed some light on what might be affecting your sleep.

As a child under five I had vivid and bizarre dreams about large human figures that would visit in a seemingly carnival type setting. The dreams would wake me up, but I'd go back to sleep. These dreams were especially full when we would visit our rustic, early 20th century summer cabin in the Santa Cruz Mountains. It was built on land next to a creek that had almost surely been lived on by Indigenous Ameri-cans. The house had the feel of many spirits, and those spirits seemed to visit me in my dreams at night. The dreams weren't so scary, but they would wake me up, and I'd lie in bed wondering what it was all about and thinking about the bizarre figures that were visiting me in my sleep.

At age six, we moved into a 1905 Spanish Style house that had been built as a country home/summer getaway in the San Francisco Mid-Peninsula area for a San Francisco family. I immediately started seeing the boogieman in the closet of my bedroom. This caused long term middle of the night scary times where I would lie awake in fear of what might be hiding in the closet. Even though I shared this room with my older brother, once awakened by the feeling of whatever was in the closet, I would lie there in fear, and it was very hard to go back to sleep.

The closet boogie-man situation morphed to anxiety about the "thousand things" that teenagers worry about, like challenges managing school homework and social situations. During the day I would self-medicate by smoking pot, but at night, I would wake up and go through the list of what I hadn't done, what I needed to do, and the thoughts about not knowing how to deal with seemingly unmanageable situations. No one ever knew any of this was going on, and it was keeping me awake for hours at a time.

Fast forward to college and the pattern of sleep issues took a new turn. A bizarre incident happened while on tour as a member of a 12-person college vocal jazz group. It involved all of us relaxing in a motel room after a concert. I was doing a neck massage, as I often did, on one of the singers, when all of a sudden, the energy got really weird in the room, and everyone got up and left. It was the room I was sharing with 3 other members of the group.

Shortly after everyone left, we all went to bed and immediately fell asleep. I started having a horrible nightmare in which I was being attacked. I startled awake, literally flew out of bed with a scream, flying over the bed next to me and then hit my mid shin on a 30-inch-high table at the front door. What ensued seemed like a reenactment of the nightmare as my three roommates stood over me confused and yelling down at me. I was terrified. Astonishingly, we all got back in bed without another word. They fell asleep, and I lay in bed thinking they were going to kill me.

This was the beginning of a recurring nightmare of being attacked through the closet, the walls, the ceiling and everything else imaginable for the next 12 years. I would startle awake, and many times think Antonia was the attacker and begin to defend myself. I would literally be in a sweat, and certainly in fight and flight, with my heart pumping and breathing fast.

I tell this story in detail, so that you can see the end result. In 1992 I returned home from a business trip abroad and developed severe gastrointestinal problems that persisted through six months of seeing GI specialists and tests to measure my digestive fluids, taking weird prescription drugs, and losing 40 pounds due to having diarrhea all the time. After all this, my doctor said, "Greg, there's nothing medically wrong with you." I left his office that day, threw the medication I was taking in the trash and drove away knowing something had to change. It was obvious I couldn't depend on other people to manage what was going on with me.

I was starving all the time due to the diarrhea, so I stopped at a new grocery store called Whole Foods. As I grazed the bread and pastry isles, I came face to face with a woman who had been a teacher in the massage certification training I had done in 1977. I looked her in the eye and said, "Priscilla, I've been meaning to call you." To my surprise she said, "I know. Your pancreas is really in trouble."

A few days later I went to her office for a 90-minute energy healing session. She called her work Bioenergy Balancing. In that 90-minute session she talked to my body, muscle tested vitamin and mineral samples, and asked my body questions about how it was or was not digesting food. She followed directions from my body about what healing was needed, traced some meridians and then asked again about my digestion.

I didn't understand what she was doing, but when I got off the table all my digestive issues were gone, completely healed, and never came back. It was an immediate change to a condition that had been chronic and unmanageable. I was very intrigued. This led to both of us becoming certified through her teaching, doing thousands of hours of apprenticing with her and starting our healing business in 1995.

Six months after that initial session I went back for what I thought would be a tune-up to make sure everything was still okay. The gastrointestinal issue was completely healed, but I was still having an occasional nightmare complete with attackers coming out of the walls yielding weapons.

As I lay on the table, a few minutes into the session, my body started to uncontrollably arch up, springing into a V shape. This happened eight or ten times accompanied by deep guttural screams. It was as if something were leaving my body. Priscilla and her co-practitioner stood on each side of me, calmly observing, until my body finally rested back down, motionless and calm. I was at peace.

What I didn't know or really understand, was that I had energetically exorcized an entity or spirit energy that had been in my body since that weird time in the motel room back in 1980. What I did know looking back a few months later, was that the nightmares were gone. Forever!

WHAT WE LEARNED

As we developed our CoreTalk Holistic Healing modality, my own case study would set the stage for a deeper understanding of how the body expresses emotional and energetic experiences through physiological conditions and symptoms to give us an understanding of how that experience is showing up in our body. Even though I didn't know exactly what experiences the energetic healing was addressing, my body was able to guide the process and heal the energetic congestion that was causing the symptoms in my body.

CLIENT CASE STUDY #1

Jane came to us in her mid-fifties after realizing she had been sexually abused as a child and through her teen years. She had been diagnosed with irritable bowel syndrome, high blood pressure, clinical depression, and obesity. Her relationship anxiety at home kept her from being able to sleep with her husband or in a bed. She had done five years of traditional talk therapy and allopathic medication before being referred to us by a friend. At her first appointment she told us about all the abuse and rape she had endured. She told us she just wanted to feel better but wasn't sure how she'd ever be able to sleep comfortably with her husband again.

In each session, we'd begin by talking with her body using muscle testing and asking yes/no questions. Her body would take us to different ages and focus on what needed to be healed from that time. She didn't remember any specifics but was sure that there had been sexual abuse throughout all ages of her youth and teen years.

We discovered that her body had energetically "split out" (clinical dissociation) hundreds, if not thousands of times throughout her childhood. The energetic splits and shock would be accompanied by adrenal fight or flight reactions, causing her body to go into adrenal overdrive. The recurring adverse childhood experiences became deeply hidden scenarios of betrayal and terror, that in adulthood, caused the chronic health conditions and made it very difficult to sleep at night.

Each time we saw Jane we would follow her body's instructions about what age it wanted to work at, the emotions it wanted to focus on, and what meridians and chakras needed attention and healing. As she began to heal the splits and bring her energy back into her body, she began to heal the chronic physical and emotional symptoms that had made going to sleep feel scary.

Over a six-month period, her digestive issues were healed, she began to feel more comfortable at work, and she was able to sleep with her husband in the same bed. This was miraculous for her as it had been years since she had had consistent sleep, much less in the same bed as her husband. She was healing the long-term effects of the thousands of ACEs she had endured in her early years.

CLIENT CASE STUDY #2

Karen is a student in our CoreTalk™ Certification Program. She is also an experienced credentialed trauma therapist. She has a long history of ACEs from family trauma in early childhood.

When she came to us, she was not sleeping well and had consistent disruptions from her three children and night owl husband. Karen found it hard to set boundaries around disruptions and tried to put up with her family's nighttime habits. The disruptions made it hard for her to go to sleep and especially hard to stay asleep.

She began clinical work with patients early in the morning and had a full schedule, many times having fully booked days with no time for self-care. To complicate matters, she had issues around food and sugar cravings that sabotaged her healthy eating plans.

During CoreTalk sessions, her body would go back to early ages between 3 and 7 years old, bringing up a wide range of emotions around traumas perpetrated by family members. Karen didn't have any clear memories of what had happened at those ages, but her body gave very specific instructions of what emotions and energetic meridians needed to be addressed and healed in regard to the traumas. She would get a great feeling of relief with each session and eventually started having less attraction to sweets and began to set boundaries with her family around what she needed for sleep.

After CoreTalk sessions, she was able to get up to 7 hours of sleep in a row. She now incorporates some energetic healing into her bedtime routine so that her body can help her with energetic balance to get consistent sleep. Doing the healing also allows her to feel empowered so she can communicate her needs with family and set boundaries around sleep without unnecessary interruptions.

WHAT WE'VE LEARNED

What we've learned in working with clients who have sleep issues is that as they begin to heal their ACEs, they begin to have better sleep. Even those with clinical insomnia and challenges with their body's systems that govern sleep (Circadian rhythms, regulation of neuro-transmitters GABA, or production of hormones like melatonin, among others), benefit from CoreTalk's ability to access and heal core issues caused from adverse experiences and emotional stress.

Dealing with and healing long term emotional stressors can be life changing, especially in regard to sleep issues. For those who have had extensive sleep issues, it may seem insurmountable, but, if you've gotten this far in the book, we have great news for you. Your sleep problem can be solved! And the even better news is that your body knows exactly what to do to heal the sleep issue and give you what you want: MORE SLEEP.

Every person's journey is different and unique. Relief can come all at once and sometimes it takes longer. What we know - after talking to thousands of bodies - is that each body has their own process, their own truth, and their own journey to sublime sleep. What we've seen is that achieving peaceful sleep, night after night, is akin to having a peaceful life, a calm mind, and a confident spirit. That is what we wish for you.

NEXT STEPS

CONGRATULATIONS ON COMPLETING GOODNIGHT, *Brain: 7 Sleep Hacks to Beat Insomnia: Go to Sleep, Get Back to Sleep, and Stay Asleep.* By implementing the sleep hacks outlined in this book and using the Good Night, Brain Sleep Log to track your progress, you've taken proactive steps towards improving your sleep quality and overall well-being.

Remember, achieving regular, restful, and rejuvenating sleep is a journey that requires dedication and consistency. As you continue to prioritize your sleep health and integrate the strategies and techniques discussed in this book into your daily routine, you'll empower yourself to overcome insomnia, reduce sleep disturbances, and enjoy the many benefits of a good night's sleep.

We encourage you to continue using the Good Night, Brain Sleep Log as a valuable tool for monitoring your sleep patterns, identifying areas for improvement, and tracking your progress over time. By regularly reviewing your sleep log and making adjustments as needed, you can cultivate healthier sleep habits and create an optimal sleep environment tailored to your needs and preferences.

As you use the Good Night, Brain Sleep Log, you can create and modify your bedtime routine as needed and move away from sleep disrupting behaviors. That way you'll be able to set and modify your sleep goals. Doing so will help you transform your sleep more quickly and easily. If, for whatever reason, you find yourself slipping back into old habits, give yourself some compassion and empathy for this beautiful transformative journey you're on. As they say, Rome wasn't built in a day, and neither was the perfect sleep schedule. Patience may sometimes be hard to come by, but it's what we need so we can continue to pursue our lifelong goal of having happy, healing, and nourishing sleep.

Thank you for embarking on this journey with us. May you continue to prioritize your sleep health, embrace restful nights, and wake up feeling refreshed, rejuvenated, and ready to take on the day. Sweet dreams and good night, brain!

LEAVE A REVIEW

If you found *Goodnight, Brain 7 Sleep Hacks to Beat Insomnia: Go to Sleep, Get Back to Sleep, and Stay Asleep* helpful in improving your sleep quality, we invite you to leave a book review on Amazon to share your experience with others. Your feedback is invaluable and can help others struggling with sleep issues discover effective strategies for achieving better sleep. If you would like to give us feedback directly, please write to us at support@selfhealthinstitute. We would love to hear from you!

DOWNLOAD THE *GOOD NIGHT, BRAIN* SLEEP MEDITATION

As a token of appreciation for your support, we've created the *Good Night, Brain* Sleep Meditation, a guided audio meditation designed to promote relaxation and prepare your mind and body for restful sleep. Click below to download your free gift and incorporate this soothing meditation into your bedtime routine for enhanced sleep quality.

www.selfhealthinstitute.com/sleepgifts

You'll also receive a free fillable .pdf copy of the Good Night, Brain

Sleep Log as our gift to you. Make sure to save a blank copy of it so you can use it again and again to address sleep issues if they come up.

BE FULL OF YOURSELF

Do you remember how we talked about being full of yourself?

Contrary to popular thought, being full of yourself is a good thing! In fact, we believe that it is pivotal to getting what you want and having a life that you love. We believe in it so much that we wrote a book about it.

Look for our upcoming book, *Be Full of Yourself*, in 2025.

CHECK OUT OUR OFFERINGS AT SELF HEALTH INSTITUTE

If you love what you see here, check out our offerings at Self Health Institute. We have many online and in person events, courses, workshops, free, fun experiences, and masterclasses that show how to heal your body, mind, and spirit in a unique and body-centric (somatic) way.

We have a CoreTalk™ Holistic Healing Certification program so you can become a certified CoreTalk™ Holistic Healing practitioner and grow a clientele of happy clients who will refer you to others every day.

Success Mastery is a Certification Program, where, over a year's time, you can learn even deeper levels of how to heal allergies, generational trauma, and chronic issues, all the while getting personal healing sessions and group calls with the two of us and our amazing certified practitioners.

Come join the fun and learn how to sweet talk your body with CoreTalk™ so that you can heal the deep, core issues that have been plaguing you for so long.

If you have issues that you haven't been able to heal, even though you have tried everything, CoreTalk™ Holistic Healing has a great track record of healing these types of issues. Write to us at support@ selfhealthinstitute.com.

ABOUT THE AUTHORS

Antonia Van Becker and Greg Lee are Master Energetic Healers who have studied sleep, meditation, energy healing, conscious breathing, Hawaiian indigenous healing, and music for decades. Since 1995, they've worked clinically in the area of the body/mind connection, natural healing, and using the body's innate healing systems to heal chronic disease, the effects of ACEs, and negative and toxic emotional settings 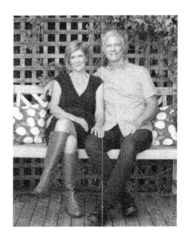 and behaviors like procrastination, self doubt, perfectionism, and limiting beliefs.

Their mission is to put healing into the hands of millions of people so they can heal themselves, their families, their pets, their friends, and their clients. This healing can then radiate throughout the world, creating a more calm and nurturing environment for all people.

As the founders of Self Health Institute, they believe that by healing old wounds and letting go of outdated beliefs and toxic relationships, we heal ourselves and create the life we've dreamed of. In doing so, the people around us, our families and our communities benefit and become part of this healing process.

For decades, Antonia and Greg have assisted people to discover and heal core issues that cause imbalance in their lives. They encourage the body's innate healing system to inform and self-heal the individual as s/he lets go of the effects of adverse experiences in mind, body, and spirit. This process is kind and loving with a spirit of loving and compassionate release.

They live in beautiful West Marin, California with their Golden Retriever, Ellie, and their Siamese Siberian Forest cat, Kona. They love to garden at Hummingbird Farm, hike, write and perform their songs.

Printed in Great Britain
by Amazon

44986031R00066